T0384853

Tie A Knot
and Hang On

SOCIAL INSTITUTIONS AND SOCIAL CHANGE
An Aldine de Gruyter Series of Texts and Monographs

SERIES EDITOR
James D. Wright, *University of Central Florida*

Thomas G. Blomberg and Stanley Cohen, **Punishment and Social Control, Enlarged Second Edition**

Rand D. Conger and Glen H. Elder, Jr., **Families in Troubled Times: Adapting to Change in Rural America**

Joel A. Devine and James D. Wright, **The Greatest of Evils: Urban Poverty and the American Underclass**

G. William Domhoff, **The Power Elite and the State: How Policy Is Made in America**

G. William Domhoff, **State Autonomy or Class Dominance: Case Studies on Policy Making in America**

Paula S. England, **Comparable Worth: Theories and Evidence**

Paula S. England, **Theory on Gender/Feminism on Theory**

R. G. Evans, M. L. Barer, and T. R. Marmor, **Why Are Some People Healthy and Others Not? The Determinants of Health of Population**

George Farkas, **Human Capital or Cultural Capital? Ethnicity and Poverty Groups in an Urban School District**

Joseph Galaskiewicz and Wolfgang Bielefeld, **Nonprofit Organizations in an Age of Uncertainty: A Study in Organizational Change**

Davita Silfen Glasberg and Dan Skidmore, **Corporate Welfare Policy and the Welfare State: Bank Deregulation and the Savings and Loan Bailout**

Ronald F. Inglehart, Neil Nevitte, Miguel Basañez, **The North American Trajectory: Cultural, Economic, and Political Ties among the United States, Canada, and Mexico**

Gary Kleck, **Targeting Guns: Firearms and Their Control**

James R. Kluegel, David S. Mason, and Bernd Wegener (eds.), **Social Justice and Political Change: Public Opinion in Capitalist and Post-Communist States**

Theodore R. Marmor, **The Politics of Medicare** (Second Edition)

Thomas S. Moore, **The Disposable Work Force: Worker Displacement and Employment Instability in America**

Clark McPhail, **The Myth of the Madding Crowd**

James T. Richardson, Joel Best, and David G. Bromley (eds.), **The Satanism Scare**

Alice S. Rossi and Peter H. Rossi, **Of Human Bonding: Parent-Child Relations Across the Life Course**

Peter H. Rossi and Richard A. Berk, **Just Punishments: Federal Guidelines and Public Views Compared**

Teresa L. Scheid, **Tie A Knot and Hang On: Providing Mental Health Care in a Turbulent Environment**

Joseph F. Sheley and James D. Wright, **In the Line of Fire: Youths, Guns, and Violence in Urban America**

David G. Smith, **Entitlement Politics: Medicare and Medicaid, 1995–2001**

David G. Smith, **Paying for Medicare: The Politics of Reform**

Linda J. Waite et al. (eds.) **The Ties That Bind: Perspectives on Marriage and Cohabitation**

Les G. Whitbeck and Dan R. Hoyt, **Nowhere to Grow: Homeless and Runaway Adolescents and Their Families**

James D. Wright, **Address Unknown: The Homeless in America**

James D. Wright and Peter H. Rossi, **Armed and Considered Dangerous: A Survey of Felons and Their Firearms** (Expanded Edition)

James D. Wright, Peter H. Rossi, and Kathleen Daly, **Under the Gun: Weapons, Crime, and Violence in America**

Tie A Knot
and Hang On

Providing Mental Health Care
in a Turbulent Environment

TERESA L. SCHEID

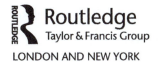

Routledge
Taylor & Francis Group

LONDON AND NEW YORK

About the Author

Teresa L. Scheid   Associate Professor, Department of Sociology, University of North Carolina at Charlotte.

First published 2004 by Transaction Publishers

2 Park Square, Milton Park, Abingdon, Oxfordshire OX14 4RN
605 Third Avenue, New York, NY 10017

Routledge is an imprint of the Taylor & Francis Group, an informa business

First issued in hardback 2020

Library of Congress Cataloging-in-Publication Data

Scheid, Teresa L.
    Tie a knot and hang on : providing mental health care in a turbulent environment / Teresa L. Scheid.
        p. cm.
Includes bibliographical references and index.
    ISBN 0-202-30758-1 (cloth : alk. paper)—ISBN 0-202-30759-X (pbk. : alk. paper)
1. Mental health services.   2. Community mental health services.
3. Mental health.   I. Title.
    RA790.S35   2004
    362.2—dc22   2003022993

ISBN 13: 978-0-202-30758-9 (hbk)

To Jeff,

with smiles and tears

Contents

Contents

Preface

Tie A Knot and Hang On is a sociological analysis of mental health care work, which crosses the borders of diverse sociological traditions. In particular, I seek to understand the theoretical and empirical linkages between environmental pressures and the activities of organizations and individuals who both enact and conform to these environmental pressures. I draw principally upon two theoretical traditions: (1) institutional theory (Scott 1995), which directs attention to the influence of institutional demands (social and normative forces) on organizational structure and behavior, and (2) emotional labor (Hochschild 1983), which focuses on the work required to create and maintain a relationship with clients. In terms of institutional theory, an important normative force is that of professionals (DiMaggio and Powell 1983). Professional norms constitute one of the primary linkages between the environment and the organization. For mental health care workers and other emotional laborers who provide care, the various feeling rules that guide their relationships with clients constitute a critical type of professional norm.

Normative beliefs and societal preferences about mental health care also constitute important institutional demands which shape the delivery of mental health care and the work of mental health care workers. The institutional demands of managed care are having a tremendous effect on the organization of mental health services and the work of mental health professionals. The institutional logic of efficiency and cost-containment conflicts with professional logics which emphasize quality care. How are mental health care organizations and providers responding to these institutional demands? How are they resolving the contradictions between different institutional demands?

While there have been many sociological studies of work in health care settings and of work in psychiatric hospitals, very few deal with the provision of community-based mental health care (but see Estroff 1981). Yet since this type of work is the ultimate exemplar of emotional labor, it is of special interest to sociologists who study work and occupations as well

as those interested in work role identity, emotional labor, and psychological burnout. Mental health care providers will also find this study helpful for understanding the larger social processes which shape their work
experiences.

Over the past ten years I have been collecting in-depth data from mental health care providers in diverse settings concerning their work and
treatment practices. I am grateful to the many providers who took time
from their busy schedules to talk with me, and who tried to show me how
their world "worked." I must also acknowledge Anselm Strauss, whose
work has served as an exemplar for my own approach to the study of mental health care. Several years ago Dr. Strauss was kind enough to review an
early draft of a paper on treatment ideology, and gave me the kind of encouraging response I needed to continue my research. Dick Scott and Karl
Weick have also provided me with positive feedback as I have struggled
to understand how mental health professionals both enact, and conform
to, institutional demands. Peggy Thoits reviewed an early draft of this
book, and provided me with excellent feedback. A number of other reviewers have helped me to clarify my arguments and I am grateful to those
colleagues, mental heath care providers and graduate students who have
read various drafts. I am honored to acknowledge the mentors and friends
who provided me with needed encouragement while I was writing this
book: Allan Horwitz, Virginia Hiday, and Bonnie Svarstad. My editors at
Aldine de Gruyter have been invaluable. I wish to thank James D. Wright
for his early encouragement, and Richard Koffler at Aldine de Gruyter for
his tireless support and timely suggestions.

I   A Sociological Analysis of Mental Health Care Workers

I've taken people to the hospital who stood at my door and cut their wrists. Once somebody went down to the Tribune with a gun and said, "I'll kill myself unless [name of clinician] talks to me on the phone." They called me and said, "You better talk to this guy," So I said to him, "Cut it out, what is this?" He gave up the gun and they brought him here to emergency and I talked to him some more. But that's typical—there are hundreds of these stories.

This was one social worker's response to my request that she describe a critical incident, that is, a story that illustrated the work of a mental health provider. The story could describe the typical types of encounters providers have with clients, or it could describe an incident that stood out in the provider's experience. The critical incident could recount a success story, or a failure. Both exemplify the work of mental health care providers. As this provider noted, the atypical is typical in this work.

The typical features of a mental health care provider's work are the focus of this book. This work involves an unusually high degree of emotional involvement with clients, which is unique and essential for the provision of mental health care. I speculate about how someone learns to deal with the kind of situation described above, especially if they must also work in public bureaucracies with too few resources and a myriad of demands from the community. These institutional demands can include increased services (from violence prevention to assisting the homeless), outreach to diverse populations (adolescents, elderly, minority groups), protection of the community from disruptive and unwanted behavior, and cost-containment. The most recent of these institutional demands is for services that are cost effective: "Managed care has burst upon the public mental health scene like a supersonic plane announced by a sonic boom" (Beigel, Minkoff, and Shore 1997: 309).

Managed care involves a fundamental change that amounts to a paradigm shift, as a rational business ethic and corresponding systems of bureaucratic control are imposed on organizations which had previously

1

operated on the basis of a professionally determined moral foundation. What happens when the emotional labor of providers is subject to increased bureaucratic scrutiny and control? Too often mental health care providers become frustrated by their work, and are no longer able to provide the kind of care they deem professionally and personally appropriate for their clients. This is the "Burned-Out Clinician." There has been an overwhelming literature on burnout in mental health care. Burned-out providers also face a series of ethical challenges as they strive to meet institutional demands for cost-containment. In the words of one provider I interviewed,

> Our society has defined success in recent times by productivity and numbers—a bottom line mentality which is often opposed to the therapeutic process and dehumanizes the clinician as well as the client.

My book is a description and a sociological analysis of mental health care work. It emphasizes the interaction of professionally generated norms which guide interactions between providers and their clients, and the organizational contexts in which care is given. Organizational settings enable, govern, and constrain these interactions. In addition, the wider social context in which mental health care is provided (referred to as the institutional environment) also constrains care, most notably by effecting the financing of care, but less obviously in influencing the very definitions of mental health and illness and the appropriate ways in which mental health providers should "treat" individuals with mental health problems.

BACKGROUND AND SIGNIFICANCE OF THE STUDY

This book builds on previous studies of medical work, which examine the interrelationship of professional, organizational, and ideological realms. Professional ideologies (or philosophies) provide meaning, context and world images (Bensman and Lilienfield 1991) as well as models of treatment and care (Abbott 1992). *Boys in White* (Becker et al. 1961: 41) studies the interrelationships between perspectives held by individuals and groups, which they defined as "the coordinated set of ideas and actions a person uses in dealing with some problematic situation." Their argument was that the behavior of medical professionals is largely a reflection of the immediate situations doctors find themselves in. Strauss et al. (1985: xi, 266) continue the tradition of the detailed "analytical examination" of medical work "within [the] thick context of organizational possibilities, constraints, and contingencies." Of critical importance are the ideological positions taken by medical workers, since their beliefs and practices affect organizational strategies for action.[1]

It is important to keep in mind that what health professionals are taught, what they learn, and what they actually practice are not entirely consistent (see Mizrahi's 1986 study of the socialization of physicians). Benner's (1984) analysis of nursing makes the distinction between practical (know-how) and theoretical (know-that) knowledge; she argues that practical knowledge is an under-researched area of clinical knowledge. Both the external context of the situation and clinician's understanding of a given situation affect the treatment choices clinicians make and their actual dealings with clients and patients. This study will examine the practical knowledge (logics in action, or knowledge in use) of front-line mental health workers, and will contribute to an understanding of the factors that influence treatment decisions and actions.

Luhrmann's (2000) ethnography of psychiatric residents provides an excellent description of the various ways treatment orientations are shaped by professional socialization. Psychiatrists approach treatment from two perspectives: either the biomedical, psycho-pharmacological or the psychodynamic psychotherapeutic. While theoretically medication and psychotherapy should be used in combination, the two approaches to treatment "are taught as different tools, based on different models, and are used for different purposes" (ibid.: 7). Furthermore, the two approaches have different organizational homes: psycho-pharmacology dominates in-patient settings where patients do not stay long enough for therapy, and psychotherapy is reserved for outpatient settings where the psychiatrist works over an extended period of time to develop a relationship with the patient. There was a happy "pluralism" between the two treatment modalities until the 1980s, when managed care entered private mental health care settings. Managed care reimburses services that have known treatment efficacy, but psychotherapy does not lend itself to the type of rigorous analysis of treatment efficacy that medication does (Horwitz 2002; Luhrmann 2000). Furthermore, prescribing medication is the one thing that psychiatrists can do that other mental health care providers cannot, and Luhrmann (2000: 99) argues that the biomedical approach is one way psychiatrists "cling to their doctorly identity" and maintain control over mental health care.

Freidson's (1986; 1989) studies of social control and the medical profession also emphasize the importance of practices and beliefs. Freidson and Abbott (1988) focus on professional conflicts, especially conflict between professional and bureaucratic authority in health care. Bureaucratic authority structures can undermine the autonomy and control of health care professionals. Central to professional status is autonomy and control over one's work. Within the mental health sector, psychiatrists and PhD psychologists are the ultimate "legitimate" professionals, traditionally wielding considerable power and authority by virtue of their expert knowledge. Social workers, therapists, and nurses are trying to gain greater professional recognition. Critical to one's relative professional status (in relation to other professionals) is the organization in which one works (Abbott 1988), and the bureaucratic or administrative control over work which can threaten or augment professional autonomy. This study will show that managed care represents an extension of bureaucratic control over clinical work and is a direct threat to the professional autonomy and discretion of providers.

Two studies of nursing demonstrate the effect of organizational contexts on care giving practices. Foner's *The Caregiving Dilemma* draws upon the literature of industrial sociology and bureaucracy to explain the working conditions of nurses' aides in long-term care facilities. She concludes that the bureaucratization of nursing home care has had the effect of "officially devaluing the supportive emotional labor nursing aids provide" (1995: 58). Chambliss (1966: 2) reveals the inherent contradiction that nurses face by being "ordered to care." Nurses are required by their job to do emotion work, yet they lack the power to decide what should be done. This contradiction is realized in the ethical dilemmas caregivers routinely face; Chambliss argues such ethical arguments are "thinly disguised turf battles" (ibid.: 8).

In a similar manner, mental health care providers experience the contradictions engendered by the commodification of care as a series of ethical dilemmas (Furman 2003; Galambos 1999; LaRoche and Turner 2002; Turney and Conway 2002). Much of this literature focuses on social workers, many of whom provide therapy in private or group practices. The central ethical dilemmas are conflicts of interest (with the provider caught between the managed care entity and the patient) and violations to confidentiality. Edwards (1999) argues that psychotherapy is no longer possible under managed care, and Galambos (1999) urges social workers to advocate for systematic reforms and equal access to mental health services. These advocacy efforts are legitimated by the ethical guidelines provided by the National Association of Social Workers.

In addition to professional domain disputes, mental health organizations also provide an excellent site for the study of different "segments," that is, those occupational groups where members share common work activities, values and identities (Halpern 1992). Abbott (1992) describes this emerging area of research as the "culture of work," and increasing attention is being given to the issue of occupational subcultures (Trice 1993). Key to any culture are the ideologies held by individuals which bind them together and help them enact their roles (Trice and Beyer 1993: 33). Different occupations and professions within an organization give rise to multiple cultures (Gregory 1983). Consequently, while there are

common orientation . . . similar problems . . . comparable experiences . . . they accommodate different beliefs and incommensurable technologies, these problems imply different solutions, and these experiences have multiple meanings. (Meyerson 1991: 131)

Mental health care providers come from many professional backgrounds. While psychiatry, psychology, social work and nursing are the most common fields (Mechanic 1999; Scott and Lammers 1985), mental health providers also have diverse backgrounds (for example religion or even sociology!). Only about one-half of mental health care providers have advanced degrees (Mechanic 1999). In addition to professional training and orientation, mental health workers are also subject to the demands of their organizational work role, which may or may not coincide with their professional background. In her study of professional groups in two psychiatric hospitals, Guy (1985) found that work setting, hierarchical rank, and tenure in the organization affected the beliefs of nurses and social workers more than professional membership. Doherty and Harry (1976) also found that organizational position (especially the shift worked) played a determinant role in shaping staff perceptions of mental patients. The specific ideological orientation to their nursing role (occupational ideology) was also found to relate to the organizations in which nurses practice (Langton 1991), providing support for Abbott's (1988) assertion that the organization in which one works is key to determining one's view of work as well as one's actual behavior. Scheid et al. (1998) in their analysis of different occupational and professional groups of mental health care providers showed that occupational identification was more important to understanding the work experiences (burnout, job satisfaction, autonomy, control) of providers than professional background.

Historically, a major divide between mental health care workers has been whether they work in the private or public sector. Those operating in the private sector operate out of office-based practices and provide therapy to clients who either pay out-of-pocket or whose care is reimbursed by private insurers. In general these clients constitute the "worried well," though clinicians in private practice also provide treatment to some individuals with serious mental illnesses. These providers typically refer to themselves as therapists.

Providers work in the public sector in large government-based agencies, serving uninsured clients and those with serious mental illnesses. Most care provided to those with serious mental illness consists of case management rather than therapy, although the extent to which therapy is integral to case management is debatable (Dill 2001). Case management involves the coordination of various services and supports (income, housing, medical care, skills training, medication, therapy) needed by the client; in addition, case managers provide emotional and tangible social support (Dill 2001). Case management may be performed by any mental health professional—nurse or social worker, psychologist or counselor. While case management may seem to be less emotionally demanding than therapy, case managers are intimately connected to their clients because they provide emotional support as well as assistance with the mechanics of living in the community. However, case management is often not deemed professionally challenging or rewarding, and may contribute to the sense of frustration that arises when individuals do not enact their role in a manner consistent with professional norms.

Dill (2001) argues that the role of the mental health case manager as gatekeeper is changing from linking clients to needed services (thereby improving access and coordination of care) to keeping costs down in the face of managed-care constraints. Case managers who are no longer able to advocate for their clients face many of the same ethical challenges as do social workers in private practice. In their ethnographic study of clinician experiences with managed care at a mental health clinic in Massachusetts, Ware et al. (2000) found that clinicians were being forced to learn a new discourse. They argue that "learning the language of managed care may mean being made over as a professional"; and report that clinicians feared they would become "the kinds of practitioners whose philosophies of treatment they deplore" (Ware et al. 2000: 19).

With managed care the divide between private practice and public sector service is becoming blurred. Managed care arrangements determine who may receive mental health care services, what types of services will be offered, and how long an individual can receive care. The treatment actions of the mental health care providers are subject to increased scrutiny and organizational control. It is likely that managed care arrangements will adversely affect the providers' input into determining organizational goals and premises for action, as well as the amounts, types, and quality of care. Services to those with chronic mental health problems are in an especially precarious position since these individuals generally require long term care or therapy as well as integrated services; yet treatment technologies do not result in proven cures (Mechanic 1994). Durham (1995: 117) notes the widespread concern that an "already vulnerable population" will be placed at "even greater risk for being managed toward the bottom line rather than toward improved client outcomes." Both public and private sector mental health care providers have been directly affected by managed care arrangements. This study addresses the changes imposed by managed care on working conditions and experiences, as well as on treatment ideologies and the provision of care.

OVERVIEW OF THEORETICAL ARGUMENT

Cost-containment, rationing of services, and performance-based outcomes characteristic of managed care are institutional demands to which mental health care organizations and providers must conform. That is, beliefs held in the wider social environment (referred to as the institutional environment) are having a direct impact on client care. Mental health care organizations have been characterized as existing in primarily institutional (as opposed to technical) environments (Hasenfeld 1992; Scott and Meyer 1991; Scott 1993). They must conform to institutional demands and beliefs about what constitutes appropriate mental health care (Scheid and Greenley 1997). The institutional environment is also the source of professional norms and practices (DiMaggio and Powell 1983) which impinge upon the daily operations of human service organizations (Hasenfeld 1992). In order to conform to professional and societal expectations, mental health organizations will change their formal structures (i.e., work arrangements and work roles). Yet mental health organizations exist in complex and turbulent institutional environments (ibid.), largely because there is little consensus among providers as to the nature of mental health and illness. As a result there is wide disagreement over the usefulness of various treatment technologies and intervention strategies as well as appropriate policy initiatives (Chandler 1990; Rochefort 1989). Mental health organizations and providers must appear to conform to a wide variety of rapidly changing and potentially contradictory institutional demands (Hasenfeld 1992; Scheid-Cook 1991). Consequently, these organizations experience "cyclical legitimacy crises" (Hasenfeld 1992: 11) and may espouse contradictory and ambiguous goals. For example, D'Aunno et al. (1991: 656) found that mental health organizations which also provide drug abuse services are characterized by "inconsistent treatment practices."

Treatment ideology is the complex set of beliefs providers hold about mental health, illness and treatment. These beliefs consist of specific theories about the etiology (i.e., the causes) of mental illness, the role of the provider and client, and the efficacy of various treatments. These sets of beliefs comprise the "feeling rules" (i.e., those norms that govern how one is supposed to feel) that providers utilize in their relationships with clients, and are critical to understanding the emotional labor of providers. Treatment ideologies will also affect organizational strategies for providing care (Strauss et al. 1985) as well as public policy (Chandler 1990; Rochefort 1989).

Treatment ideologies are not an individual's beliefs or opinions; rather they are collective in nature and serve to legitimate existing ways of doing things. The collective site of treatment ideologies is the organizations where providers meet, learn and work (as illustrated so well by Luhrmann's [2000] study of psychiatric residents). Ideologies bind people together via common beliefs (i.e., culture) and help them enact their roles within the organization (Trice and Beyer 1993). While treatment ideologies are central features of an organization's culture, they arise from past experiences, training, and concrete work experiences and are reproduced, modified, or changed by the current organization in which a provider works. One of the critical issues is whether managed mental health care will limit the power and autonomy of mental health care providers by imposing organizational constraints on treatment.

Studies have shown that organizational context affects treatment offerings (Holland et al. 1981; Mechanic 1976; Morrissey et al. 1984; O'Driscoll and Evans 1988; Prager 1986). In their analysis of the mental health industry in the 1970s, Magaro et al. (1978) found that treatments (service offerings) followed from cultural conceptions of madness which were expressed in the beliefs of mental health personnel. They found that different organizational systems (administrative versus professional) reflected different sets of professional and cultural beliefs about treatment (control versus treatment). Yet few studies examine the ways in which the ideological positions of mental health workers affect organizational strategies (Strauss et al. 1985).

Organizations incorporate social and professional beliefs into their culture, or definition of reality, via complex processes of enactment (Daft and Weick 1984; Weick 1977). Enactment involves the active construction (creation) of the information to which the organization responds. That is, organizations choose their environments (or particular normative prescriptions) which then become extensions of the organization (Morgan 1986). Organizations do not merely adopt (or avoid) external constraints or normative prescriptions; they first must create the perception that an external pressure requires some action. As Weick describes the process, "people, often alone, actively *put* things out there that they then perceive and negotiate about perceiving" (1979: 165).

I found a great deal of variability in the ways in which mental health organizations responded to and used outpatient commitment as a legal tool to enforce community-based treatment. Some organizations did not use outpatient commitment at all, and those that did exhibited tremendous variability in the procedures and means for handling their clients despite the fact that outpatient commitment was a "clear-cut" legal policy with specific rules.[2] I found that professional ideologies and organizational beliefs about treatment were critical to the ways in which the mental health centers "enacted" outpatient commitment (Scheid-Cook 1992). Those that adhered to a biomedical view of mental illness and treatment used outpatient commitment as a mechanism to keep clients on medication. Mental health organizations in which community-based care was primary also used outpatient commitment as a means to keep in close contact with clients. Those organizations that were more concerned with social control of clients generally did not use outpatient commitment; instead they relied upon the traditional route of re-hospitalization via civil commitment to control noncompliant clients. Other organizations did not use outpatient commitment because they felt it represented an implicit means of social control and force, which conflicted with treatment ideologies that emphasized patient liberty and empowerment. Thus treatment ideology is critical in understanding how organizations interpret and enact institutional demands which exist outside the organization.

In addition to social beliefs and professional ideologies, organizations themselves may also be a significant source of treatment ideologies. This is because providers do their work in organizations, and theoretical belief systems are shaped and modified by practical work experiences (Benner 1984). Specific organizational structures and the availability of resources will limit the range of treatment ideologies that can be implemented in a given organization. In his classic study of mental hospitals, Perrow (1965) found that the cultural system (i.e., the institutional environment) established two legitimate goals for mental hospitals: custodial care and therapeutic care. Yet the authoritarian structure of the hospital was consistent only with custodial goals because an adequate technology to meet treatment goals was lacking. Similarly, community mental health centers in the 1980s lacked the means to provide for those with chronic mental illnesses in the community (Chandler 1990; Horwitz 1987; Lamb 1982). Strauss et al. (1964: 360) argued that ideologies are mediated by operational philosophies which are "systems of ideas and procedures for implementing therapeutic ideologies under specific institutional conditions." That is, what one would ideally like to do, or feel one ought to do (fundamental aspects of the organization's ideology) and what one can realistically do in a given organization (the operative aspects) may well conflict (Abravanel 1983). For example, ideally and fundamentally, treatment for a client with a chronic mental illness calls for effective cures and the client's return to a "normal" life via skills training, vocational rehabilitation, and ongoing social supports. Realistically and operatively, medication maintenance may be all that can be done with existing resources.

However, individuals in organizations have many strategies for managing the conflicts that arise between the fundamental and operative aspects of the organizational ideology, the most important of which are the mediatory myths (Abravanel 1983; Scheid-Cook 1988). Myths not only presuppose the validity of a particular belief or practice, but they also prevent individuals from directly acknowledging ideological contradictions. Mental health providers must maintain confidence in their work; they must believe that what they are doing does make a difference; that what they *can* do (operative actions) contributes to what *should* be done (fundamental beliefs). Obviously fundamental beliefs are analogous to the feeling rules which characterize the emotional labor of providers.

In research on outpatient commitment in the 1980s I found that beliefs about medication were mediatory myths central to the ideology of mental health providers (Scheid-Cook 1988). Believing that medication is the principal component of outpatient treatment allowed providers to get on with their work despite the contradictions between the ideal of maintaining clients in the community without adequate community supports. Specifically, providers felt that outpatient commitment could help them keep clients on medication following discharge from the hospital; if the clients could "be maintained" on medication long enough, they might exhibit "medication compliance" and gain "insight" into their mental illness. The myth holds that once clients gain "insight" they will understand why continued medication is necessary for remaining in the community and staying out of the hospital. Once such insight is reached, other forms of treatment (psychotherapy or skills training) can be utilized. Medication also forms a bridge between the ideal of treatment as a "cure" and the reality that "most of them will never get better." By believing in the efficacy of medication, providers can overcome the contradictions between the fundamental and operative goals of the organization, as well as resolve conflicting institutional purposes (i.e., social control versus therapy). This is not to say all providers believe in the efficacy of medication, but that the treatment ideology exhibited by many mental health organizations in the 1980s emphasized medication compliance as a means to community stability. Similarly, mediatory myths play an important role in reconciling conflict between competing institutional demands for cure as opposed to care, and for cost-containment as opposed to quality care.

Managed care represents a response to the wider normative demand for technical rationality and efficiency. Meyer (1990) conceptualizes this process of rationalization in terms of the commodity model of organizations (in contrast to the traditional bureaucratic model). Rationality is not so much a matter of finding the appropriate means to a given end (the bureaucratic model), but of achieving given ends—the accumulation of wealth, profit, or saving public monies (the commodity model). In terms of mental health care services, the institutional expectation is that certain kinds of delivery systems or treatment practices will produce specific mental health care outcomes. Organizations and providers must be concerned with meeting goals of cost-containment (whether for profit-based systems or to save "scarce" public dollars), determining the most effective means to achieve these financially determined goals, and then monitoring performance to ensure that services are delivered in a cost-efficient manner (Flood and Fennel 1995).

Because of these institutional demands for efficiency (in the name of commodification), the discipline and control of all professional groups has been undergoing formalization and centralization. The literature on professional power has traditionally focused on the conflict between bureaucratic and professional power, and has shown that the decline in professional power involves deprofessionalization (loss of trust in professional prerogative), proletariatization (loss of autonomy and skill discretion), or corporatization (Wolinsky 1993). Most studies of managed care emphasize deprofessionalization, either in terms of patients' loss in trust in their health care providers (Mechanic and Schlesinger 1996) or physician's loss of autonomy due to mechanisms put in place by managed care (Schlesinger and Gray 1997). I argue that the institutional logic of commodification conflicts directly with professionally-based logics of mental health care. Light (1997) has analyzed the commodification of health care as a movement from a provider-driven to a buyer-driven system. In provider-driven health care, professionals maintained control over decisions about appropriate care, and their primary focus was on quality care. Scott et al. (2000) term the provider-driven system as the era of professional dominance. It was the dominant logic until the early 1980s. With the "buyers revolt" (Light 1997), health care has moved to a system characterized by a distrust of professional authority, a focus on external accountability and monitoring, and the rise of corporate health care systems. The era of managed care values cost-containment above quality care, although there have been efforts to implement quality-based performance indicators.

Consistent with Freidson's (1984) argument that the profession will continue to exercise control over their professional work is the evidence that physicians have maintained clinical authority over treatment decisions, although they also incorporate principles of cost-containment into their professional logics. However, we do not know how health care providers who do not have the expertise and training of physicians will fare when confronted with powerful demands for efficiency and cost-containment. It is more likely that professional logics of care (i.e., treatment ideologies) will be co-opted or ultimately displaced by forces propelling commodification.

One effect of conformity to diverse institutional demands is increased intraorganizational diversity. That is, a greater variety of professionals will be hired to fill the diverse needs of the organization (i.e., drug abuse specialists as well as therapists; utilization reviewers as well as case managers). This situation can result in higher levels of interprofessional conflict, as well as greater ambiguity over appropriate treatment ideologies. Conflicting institutional demands are mirrored within the organization by differing treatment ideologies that in practice can result in diverse and uncoordinated service offerings. Providers are more likely to experience frustration and burnout as they attempt to shift through contradictory feeling rules and standards for practice. This situation is amplified within the wider rubric of managed care; providers must make difficult choices between their own professional beliefs about necessary care and organizationally mandated constraints on that care, which are attempts to meet institutional demands for efficiency.

In addition to providing an analysis of how institutional demands and organizational conditions affect treatment practices, this book also provides a sociological analysis of psychological burnout. Burnout refers specifically to the emotional and physical depletion associated with conditions of work in human service organizations (Farber 1983; Jackson et al. 1986; Starrin et al. 1991). Researchers and mental health providers have targeted the organization as the source of burnout, attributing it to role overload, role conflict, and role ambiguity, or lack of supervisory support (Cherniss 1980; Jayaratne and Chess 1983; Latack 1986; Motowildo et al. 1986; Schulz et al., 1995; Wolpin et al. 1991). Others point to the clients, especially those with severe, persistent mental illnesses who are especially needy, as the primary "cause" of burnout (Atwood 1982; Lang 1981; Stern and Minkoff 1979). Clients with severe mental illnesses show little evidence of concrete gains or improvement; in fact, they may not even agree that they have any particular problem that needs clinical attention, and this can thwart efforts of the mental health worker. Indeed, many of the providers in private practice I interviewed left the public sector because they burned out working with so many needy clients.

Rather than targeting the organization (many of us work in stressful environments) or the client as the source of burnout, I argue that burnout is endemic to mental health providers because their work involves emotional labor. It is not the lack of resources, or the lack of community support, nor is it the difficult and oftentimes recalcitrant client, or the bureaucratic working conditions that *cause* burnout. While burnout is certainly exacerbated by stressful working conditions, it is distinguished by the factor of emotional labor, which requires an investment of self into one's work in order to maintain the necessary therapeutic relationship. This "work" involves building and maintaining relationships with many clients, and can produce a sense of both personal and professional accomplishment, but it can also produce the symptoms of burnout: emotional exhaustion, depersonalization (or cynicism) and a notable lack of personal accomplishment.

Emotional labor occurs when "the emotional style of offering the service is part of the service itself" (Hochschild 1983: 5). Emotional labor has been commonly associated with service work, or work that involves interactions with clients, and it occurs when work involves dealing with others' feelings in addition to the regulation of one's own feelings (James 1989). Luhrmann (2000: 67) describes the emotional labor of psychotherapists who learn to "be deeply, emotionally engaged with their patients, and yet not respond to their own needs."

Emotional labor involves both *surface acting* (where workers display emotions they do not necessarily feel) and *deep acting* (where the worker actually feels the emotions expressed and must therefore invest more of themselves into the work role). The emotional labor produced by mental health care workers is typical of deep acting, where mental health care workers draw upon emotional memory and actually experience the emotion they are required to display with clients (i.e., concern, regret, empathy). Mental health care workers (and other health care providers) are caregivers who must respond emotionally to their clients. Himmelweit

(1999) argues that caring work must be distinguished from other jobs involving emotional labor by the fact that emotional labor is not a cost, but a desirable aspect of the job (see also Treweek 1996). "Caregiving is a balancing act of attachment to and detachment from others" (Kahn 1993: 554); mental health care demands that providers develop and maintain meaningful relationships. Mental health care providers must learn the appropriate feeling rules in order to fulfill the emotional demands of their caring roles. If they become overinvolved with clients (a lack of detachment) or too detached (hardened and cynical) they risk psychological burnout and will be less competent caregivers. Professional norms specify the appropriate feeling rules as well as providing some guidance about how to avoid burnout—the negative consequences of emotional labor.

Standards governing emotional labor are professionally and occupationally dictated, and organizational working conditions can hinder or assist one's ability to perform emotional labor. Consequently, burnout must be understood in terms of a complex interaction between professional standards, occupational norms, and organizational contexts which influence job performance and affect identity. The profession dictates the appropriate feeling rules for performance of one's work, which in the case of the mental health care provider is the development and maintenance of a therapeutic relationship. Both professional socialization and occupational experience help shape work identity, which includes treatment ideology. Treatment ideology consists of the specific beliefs about the etiology of mental illness, the role of the provider and the client, the goals of treatment, and the efficacy of various treatments. Treatment ideologies are therefore critical referents for action; they contain the feeling rules which dictate the specific type of emotional labor required in the therapeutic relationship.

Yet the organization, the insurer, or a supervisor may assume varying degrees of control over the ways in which emotional workers will enact their professional work roles. Sociologists have long studied the various ways in which organizations seek to control labor (both emotional and physical) and limit the autonomy and decision making input of their employees (Berger et al. 1973; Hochschild 1983; Leidner 1993; Schwalbe 1986). The critical organizational conditions of work which contribute to burnout are those which affect one's work identity and subsequently one's sense of personal accomplishment. The organization can help the worker to manage the difficult demands of emotional labor successfully, or it can make this task nearly impossible via the speed-up (too many clients or increased caseloads), bureaucratic demands (priority placed on paperwork or utilization review), role ambiguity or conflict, a difficult supervisor or poor relations with supervisors. These conditions can, in and of themselves, produce stress, but the unique requirements of emotional labor produce the conditions necessary for burnout.

RESEARCH OBJECTIVES

This book analyzes the ways in which shifting institutional frameworks shape mental health care and the work of mental health care providers. In Chapter 2 I examine how etiologies of mental illness (beliefs about the causes of mental illness) are shaped by larger social beliefs, priorities, and expectations about mental health care. I describe the movement of mental health care systems from institutional to community-based care. Etiologies of illness are clearly related to different institutional environments, and ultimately influence the treatment practices and ideologies of health care providers. Chapter 2 also describes conflicting etiologies of mental illness, and providers' views and understandings about the sources of mental illness. These etiologies are critical to understanding treatment ideologies, which are the focus of Chapter 3. That chapter develops a typology of treatment ideologies and examines the degree of consistency of treatment ideologies within two public sector mental health care organizations. I investigate the extent to which treatment ideologies are widely shared by providers, and the degree to which treatment ideologies have changed in response to new institutional demands for care.

Chapters 4 and 5 focus on the new institutional demand for managed care and cost-containment, and raise the following questions: What effect has managed care had on mental health care? How has it changed the work role of providers? Do providers have less control and autonomy? Have mental health care providers faced the ethical challenges outlined in the literature? Chapter 4 focuses on providers in the private sector while Chapter 5 analyzes the ways in which managed care has changed the service offerings of one public sector agency. If left unchecked, managed care has the potential to greatly decrease the control and decision-making latitude of providers, and to increase the extent of psychological demands placed upon providers (via the speed-up of seeing too many clients in too little time) while also setting limits on the types of emotional labor providers are able to perform (i.e., limiting visits, emphasizing short-term therapies and medications). Consequently, mental health care work will be less fulfilling and providers will experience a diminished sense of professional accomplishment.

Chapter 6 analyzes the relationship between emotional labor and burnout in depth. I argue that work identity is crucial to understanding burnout, and that the work identity of providers consists of feeling rules which govern relationships with clients (and which comprise the treatment ideologies of providers). This chapter describes the emotional labor of providers and analyzes the relationship between emotional labor, working conditions and burnout. Chapter 7 describes the effect that managed care has had on the emotional labor of providers and the various ways in which managed care has exacerbated their stress and burnout.

In Chapter 8 I return to the institutional environment and examine those emerging institutional forces which will shape mental health care in the future, with a focus on forces that will limit the potential abuses of managed care. First I examine various efforts to reconcile the conflict between professional logics and the logic of cost-containment that characterize an ideology of public sector managed care. I demonstrate that an important institutional demand is for quality care, and describe various efforts to implement standards for quality care. Second I examine the movement to privatize public mental health services and point out that policy advocates constitute an institutional force. I also describe the impact of the National Alliance for the Mentally Ill (NAMI) and the National Mental Health Association (NMHA) have on mental health care. In Chapter 9 I consider the future of mental health care, and include descriptions in the providers' own words.

SOURCES OF EVIDENCE

As a graduate student I had a primary role in the collection of data on the effects of deinstitutionalization on individuals with severe mental illnesses, as part of a large statewide study that focused on client outcomes. Given my concentration in organization sociology I quickly became interested in how mental health care had changed in response to changing institutional demands. My dissertation focused upon outpatient commitment, a policy which provides for the court-ordered involuntary treatment of individuals in the community on an outpatient basis. The articles published from the dissertation analyzed outpatient commitment in terms of contradictory institutional demands (Scheid-Cook 1988, 1991), organizational enactments of institutional demands (Scheid-Cook 1992), and outpatient commitment as a form of social control (Scheid-Cook 1991, 1993). In the course of two years of data collection (including four organizational case studies) I interviewed many mental health providers about their work with clients. These were informal, conversational interviews that utilized questions from Schatzman and Strauss's (1973) *Health Professional Interview*. I became interested in mental health work, and have continued to interview providers. The interview protocol has been modified over the years, and includes questions from Benner's (1984) study of nursing. Providers are asked to describe a critical incident, a typical day at work and an unusual day at work. I have also added questions about burnout and managed care. The interview took about an hour, and providers seemed to enjoy the opportunity to discuss their work. My interviews with providers were among the most delightful hours I have spent as a researcher.

In the early 1990s I collected data from a large public mental health center which provides services in an urban Standard Metropolitan Statistical

Area (SMSA; this data site will be referred to as CARE).[3] At that time, CARE employed over seventy primary care clinicians who provided coordinated case management to clients with severe mental illnesses. Caseloads ranged from thirty to thirty-five clients, though providers worked in teams and had team support to help them manage these large caseloads. I selected a stratified random sample of providers (stratified on the basis of occupational category) and contacted twenty-four providers for an interview. Of that group, twenty-two providers were able to complete the interview (two did not have enough time). In addition to the qualitative interviews, I attended ten retreats held with the different treatment teams and medical service units at CARE.

I have continued to collect data from CARE, which now provides services to over 1,500 clients with severe, chronic mental illnesses. CARE began planning for a movement to managed care in 1996 and hired a Managed Care Director to develop and implement a strategy to manage care. I interviewed directors and administrators responsible for implementing managed care, and attended staff meetings and development meetings with groups of providers. My role has been that of a nonparticipant observer, and I am a familiar and accepted presence at the organization. In the spring of 1998 I distributed a questionnaire to all direct care providers (n = 90) in order to collect data on the organization prior to managed care. The questionnaire was replicated in 2000 in order to evaluate the impact of managed care. The response rate in 1998 was 56.6 percent (n = 51), and in 2000 it was 49 percent (n = 46). There was tremendous turnover in those two years; with forty-nine providers leaving the organization.

In terms of their orientation to community-based care, CARE is remarkably similar to a sample of nineteen mental health outpatient programs studied in Wisconsin (Scheid and Greenley 1997); although CARE places greater emphasis on substance abuse services. The scales assessing working conditions and experiences (work environment, autonomy, satisfaction, job involvement, and psychological burnout) are also similar. Despite the fact the CARE "looks" like other community mental health care centers, it is unique in its proactive movement toward managed care, and its attempt to preserve the ideology of community based care as well as professional control of mental health care services. In addition, CARE is unique in that it is the first public sector agency to obtain accreditation from the National Committee for Quality Assurance (NCQA). Consequently, CARE is a substantively as well as theoretically significant case, and warrants in-depth study (Berg 1990; Ragin 1999). Health services research has suffered from a premature focus on large-scale studies (where diversity makes any kind of generalization difficult) and a dearth of empirically grounded case study research (Devers et al. 1999). Thus this study makes an important contribution to the research literature on managed care.

I also interviewed fourteen other providers at a second public mental health center, located in a midsized city in another state. SUPPORT is somewhat smaller than CARE, and more decentralized, with five separate Community Support Programs that provide community outreach to clients. At the time I collected data SUPPORT employed forty primary care providers. A team model was utilized in which clinicians had caseloads of twelve to fifteen, yet also provided team support to another twenty clients.

CARE and SUPPORT provide primarily case management; both organizations are widely regarded as being highly innovative and successful, and deeply committed to the delivery of quality mental health care to individuals with severe mental illnesses. The major difference in organizational role structure is that at SUPPORT the nurses (mostly RNs) were also case managers and each treatment team had at least one nurse who administered medication. At CARE nurses worked out of a separate medication unit. They were organized into teams and did not perform any case management duties. Consequently they did not have caseloads but instead provided medication and worked closely with psychiatrists and case managers to coordinate medication and supportive services. Providers at SUPPORT also completed the questionnaire.

Table 1 contains demographic information on the providers who were interviewed, compared to those who completed the written questionnaire. The gender and race composition of the respondents corresponds to the overall demographic composition at the respective sites. The bachelor's degree is the terminal degree for one-half of the clinicians at CARE, with another fourth having a master's degree and one-fourth with some other degree (generally nursing). Clinicians at SUPPORT had higher levels of professional training, with the majority possessing the master's degree, generally in social work. In terms of organizational work role, the majority of those interviewed at both sites were case managers; a proportionate number also had some supervisory responsibilities for their unit or treatment team. At both sites, the clinical coordinator was included in the in-depth interviews.

In the summer of 1998 I also conducted a case study analysis of a private, non-profit mental health care agency which provides training to psychiatric residents and which implemented a managed care system in 1989. This agency—located in the same state as SUPPORT but in a different city—holds the county contract for Medicaid clients and exemplifies the privatization of public sector care which results from managed care. My research consisted of interviews with administrators and key staff as well as focus group interviews with case managers and social workers.

In order to study the effect of managed care on private sector mental health work, I began interviewing private clinicians in the late 1990s. I utilized the *Directory of Professional Members* developed by the Mental Health Association in the urban SMSA where CARE is located.[4] The directory

Table 1. Demographic Background of Providers in Public Sector (%)

	CARE			SUPPORT	
	Interview (N=22)	1998 Survey (N=51)	2000 Survey (N=46)	Interview (N=14)	Survey (N=41)
GENDER					
Male	27%	24%	30%	57%	46%
Female	73	76	70	43	54
RACE					
White	64	64	60	100	96
Black	36	36	40	—	4
EDUCATION					
BA—Psychology	27	33	30	0	8
BA—Other	27	20	11	0	17
MA/MSW	23	25	33	86	58
PhD/MD	0	0	0	0	0
Nursing	23	22	26	14	17

listed forty-one private mental health providers; I selected a stratified sample (stratified by gender and professional degree) of fifteen providers to interview in-depth. Eleven interviews were completed (for a response rate of over 70 percent); once again providers were willing to be interviewed and enjoyed the time talking about their work. Table 2 contains information about the private providers whom I interviewed; they are in general representative of the population frame. All were white, 64 percent were women, and close to one-half had a MSW. Unlike providers in the public sector, all of the private clinicians had an advanced degree with specialized clinical training. In order to pretest the instrument and to check on the generalizability of the information obtained in the personal interviews, another nine providers completed a written questionnaire that contained an equal number of open-ended and fixed-choice questions about their work and the effects of managed care.

In the fall of 1998 22 providers in private practice completed the questionnaire (with a response rate of 46 percent). The same sampling list was utilized, and there was considerable turnover in the listing of professionals. The 1998 Directory contained 48 providers, 25 of whom were listed in both the 1997 and 1998 Directories. Ten providers who were listed in 1997 were no longer in the Directory; the majority of whom I determined via follow-up had left their private practices. Another 31 providers had added their names to the Directory, generally in hope of obtaining additional clients.

Table 2. Demographic Background of Providers in Private Practice (%)

	1997 Directory (N=41)	Personal Interview (N=11)	1998 Directory (N=48)	Completed Questionnaire (N=22)
GENDER				
Male	44%	36%	48%	41%
Female	56	64	52	59
EDUCATION				
MA	22	0	16.7	22.7
MSW	39	63	20.8	22.7
PhD	32	27	54.2	50.0
MD	7	9	8.3	4.6

I utilize the model for grounded theory presented by Glaser and Strauss (1967) and Strauss and Corbin (1990) to analyze the qualitative data. The data are coded by recurrent themes, referred to as categories, and the various dimensions of the conceptual categories. For example, burnout is a critical conceptual category that contains many subdimensions (i.e., definitions of burnout, sources of burnout, consequences of burnout) which are central to this analysis. In order to elaborate or explicate the relationship between key concepts coded in the data, theoretical (or analytical) memos were written. Qualitative data allow for the generation of new knowledge and hypotheses; it is less useful for testing research hypotheses. The generalizability of the concepts, rather than the findings, is the primary strength of grounded theory (Conrad 1990). When I began collecting data on the work of providers, I did not realize the importance of emotional labor, and did not even consider mental health work from this perspective. In analyzing the data emotional labor emerged as a critical component of mental health work, and a potential source of burnout. Qualitative data give a fuller sense of the nature of emotional labor and burnout than quantitative data alone. A preliminary paper describing my analysis of burnout and organizational working conditions was made available to the providers whom I interviewed so that they might correct any inaccuracies and provide feedback.

In developing my arguments I rely heavily on qualitative data; quantitative data are used to confirm the results of the qualitative analysis. Qualitative data used to describe the experiences of providers are representative and convey their collective story. Quotes from individual clinicians exemplify common experiences and general themes. Consequently, I do not try to identify individual providers beyond noting their occupational roles and whether they are in public or private practice, where this information is appropriate and useful. Providing more information would individualize their accounts in such a way as to undermine the investigator's ability to generalize from their experiences and might compromise their confidentiality.

NOTES

1. It is interesting that Strauss et al. (1985: 284) refer indirectly to Karl Weick's concept of organizational enactment when they conceive of the environment "as literally inside the organization itself, in the form of workers carrying the outside into the work of the organization."

2. Obviously no legal policy is "clear-cut"; all are subject to interpretation and negotiation. Yet the outpatient commitment law was reasonably short, concise, and specific.

3. I will provide only minimal details about the mental health centers where I collected my data in order to protect their anonymity.

4. This Directory is viewed as an excellence reference guide to private mental health care providers in this city. The Mental Health Association solicits information from all licensed private providers and asks them to provide detailed information on their educational background, certifications, areas of specialty, hospital affiliations, and managed care contracts. I believe (as does the president of the MHA) that the Directory contains a listing of the most professional and conscientious private mental health care providers.

2   Reluctant Managers

The Treatment of Mental Illness

A person with a mental disability has a piece of their life that is just a little out of whack, a bit. I really believe there is more in common with me and a person with mental illness than there are differences. (Female case manager)

I think it's a biological illness. I think it's mainly a chemical thing. Clearly it's a combination of a lot of factors: social, psychological. It's amazing how complex it is. How incredibly diverse everybody is. (Female nurse case manager)

In this chapter I examine how providers view their clients[1] and focus on the different etiologies of mental illness and the implications of these etiologies for client care and treatment. As the above quotations exemplify, providers' views about the nature of mental illness are contradictory and controversial, and lead to a good bit of ambiguity over appropriate treatment initiatives. No one chooses to be a mental health care client; mental illness is one of the most stigmatizing of illnesses. The label "mentally ill" confers a master status that overrides other personality traits and assigns the individual a spoiled identity (Goffman 1961). Consequently, individuals are reluctant to seek help even when faced with fairly "normal" periods of emotional distress (such as after a divorce). Many of the providers described in this book work primarily with one of the most difficult client populations, namely, those with severe, persistent mental illnesses. These clients provide little evidence of concrete gains or improvements, and often do not cooperate with treatment recommendations. Consequently, as one public sector provider stated, "no one wants our clients." The emphasis on case management and the provision of social supports force providers in the public sector to become "managers" rather than "therapists." This shift represents a movement to a biopsychosocial as opposed to a medical or psychosocial model of mental illness. With managed care, the conflict between psychosocial and medical views of treatment plays out in a new institutional framework which authorizes care based upon medical necessity.

21

These shifts in preferences for care reflect changes in the wider institutional environment, social beliefs, priorities, and expectations (i.e., institutional demands) about mental health care. Beliefs about mental illnesses also influence people's willingness to seek help. Consequently, I begin this chapter with a brief review of mental health care in the United States, describing the movement from institutional to community-based services. I then describe the conflicting etiologies of mental illness and the providers' views and understandings about the sources of mental illness. The majority of providers I interviewed regard mental illness in terms of an integrated biopsychosocial model. In the final section of the chapter I delineate how the mental health sector changed to conform to institutional demands for community-based care that is founded on a biopsychosocial perspective of mental health.

MODELS OF MENTAL HEALTH CARE

The types of services available to those with mental health problems are shaped by widely held values and beliefs about mental health and illness. There have been four major phases of care, each of which reflects different societal values, political preferences, and economic priorities (Scheid 1999): First, the phase of institutionalized care, which was dominant from the late 1800s until the mid-1900s, during which the primary locus of care was the mental hospital. Second, the phase of deinstitutionalization that emerged in the 1950s and began to recede in the mid-1980s, and was typified by the closing of state hospitals and movement of patients into the community. Third, the consolidation of community-based care that took place during the 1980s and into the 1990s, which was characterized by efforts to coordinate and integrate community services as well as to extend services to those in need. I will only provide a brief description of each of these three phases; see Grob (1994) for more complete descriptions and analyses. The fourth phase, to be described more fully later, is the movement to managed care. Managed care is reshaping both the private and public mental health sectors, and is characterized by a technocratic rationality with a concomitant emphasis upon cost-containment and efficiency.

During the institutionalization phase, most care and treatment of those with mental illnesses took place in private or large state hospitals. A type of moral therapy (Morrissey et al.1980) prevailed in the early nineteenth century, which was reflected in the mental hygiene movement. Mental illness was not seen as a disease, but as undesirable behavior that could be changed (Torrey 1988). Treatment was largely provided by psychiatrists, who had an extensive role to fulfill. As cited in Torrey (1988: 48), the psychiatrist "has not only to be the diagnostician and the prescriber of drugs and diet, or surgery and mechanical therapeutics, but he has to be the educator and instructor of his patients."

Mental hospitals are "total institutions" (Goffman 1961) that provide for all of the patient's needs (housing, food, treatment, medical care, social interaction) in a highly regimented and controlled environment. Goffman (ibid.: 352) describes the prevailing treatment ideology in terms of the medical service model which served to meet institutional demands for custodial care:

> Part of the official mandate of the public mental hospital is to protect the community from the danger and nuisance of certain kinds of misconduct. In terms of the law and of the public pressures to which the mental hospital is sensitive, this custodial function is of major importance.

While the diagnosis of mental illness generally was based on some form of medical criteria, treatment was largely custodial (as opposed to therapeutic). Furthermore, because of the involuntary nature of most commitments to the hospital, as well as the small numbers of mental health professionals dealing with increasingly large patient populations, custodial care became a matter of social control, as depicted in Ken Kesey's novel, *One Flew Over the Cuckoo's Nest* (1962).

Deinstitutionalization was in part a response to the wider critique that hospitals were merely warehouses for those who were unwanted in the community. The movement of individuals from the hospital to the community reflected both social and professional preferences for greater individual liberty and less structured treatment settings. Outpatient care became the preferred treatment modality, with a concurrent emphasis upon normalization and adjustment. However, deinstitutionalization was also propelled by changes in the financing of mental health care. New sources of public funding at the federal level for community mental health centers and the extension of welfare benefits to those with mental illnesses allowed community-based care to become a reality. The segregative social control provided by the state hospital had simply became too costly to maintain (Scull 1977), and those with severe mental illnesses were returned to the community where costs were lower. At the same time, the advent of psychotropic drugs provided the technological means to allow for community-based care. As a result, over 400,000 patients were released from the late 1950s to the early 1980s and communities scrambled to find places for them. Many ended up homeless (Torrey 1988).

In place of state hospitals, the Community Mental Health Centers (CMHC) Act of 1963 directed each state to develop a plan designating catchment areas that would serve 75,000 to 200,000 people who would be served by a community mental health center.[2] The CMHC was designed to provide social supports in the community, and reflected a social rather than a medical model of illness. Community mental health centers were intended to develop the adaptive capacities of the client and promote community integration, while at the same time fostering community attitudes of tolerance, respect, and helpfulness toward the client (Bockoven 1972). While psychiatric medication controls some of the more overt symptoms of mental illness, individuals with chronic mental illnesses face certain functional limitations that prevent their successful integration into the community. In resident household data collected in 1989 by the National Center for Health Statistics, close to half of those with serious mental illness between the ages of 18 and 69 were unable to work, and another 52.6 percent had trouble coping with day-to-day stress (National Center for Health Statistics, Advance Data No. 218; September 16, 1992).

However, CMHCs were criticized for serving primarily the "worried well"—those with less acute disorders and excluding those with chronic and severe illnesses from their institutions. At the same time, communities did not accept individuals with severe illnesses; and so community integration and normalization remained a chimera. Community mental health centers were inadequately funded, and mental health providers were not initially prepared to deal with the diverse needs of those with chronic mental illness. Most mental health professionals had been trained to do psychotherapy, and individuals with chronic mental illnesses were seen by many as being among the least desirable type of client (Atwood 1982; Lang 1981; Stern and Minkoff 1979).

The consolidation of community-based care utilized a variety of mechanisms to improve the delivery of outpatient care to those with severe, persistent mental illnesses. People with chronic mental illnesses need a wide variety of social supports to survive in the community, and they require ongoing or long-term care, and the CMHCs were criticized for failing to provide or coordinate the necessary support services for such care (Mechanic and Rochefort 1990; Shadish et al. 1989). However, funding for community-based care began to decline in the 1980s with Reagan's Omnibus Reconciliation Act of 1980, resulting in various strategies to integrate existing services. Care was coordinated at the individual level by case management and multidisciplinary treatment teams, at the organizational level by the development of Community Support Programs, and at the service system level by the development of mental health authorities. These mechanisms for coordinated care will be described more fully later in this chapter. At this point, I will discuss the medical and social models of mental illness, and describe provider views of mental illness.

UNDERSTANDING MENTAL ILLNESS

The most recent national epidemiological study of the prevalence of mental illness in the community, the National Comorbidity Survey, interviewed 8,028 individuals in 1991 (in thirty states) and reported that 49.7 percent of those surveyed reported one lifetime episode of psychiatric disorder; 30.9 percent had one or more disorders in the twelve months immediately prior to the interview (Kessler and Zhao 1999). The most common disorders assessed in the National Comorbidity Survey were major depression and alcohol dependence. Seventeen percent of the respondents reported an episode of major depression in their lifetime; 10 percent reported an episode within the past twelve months. Fourteen percent of the respondents had a lifetime history of alcohol dependence, with 7 percent dependent in the last year. Women were more likely to experience an episode of major depression and men were more likely to experience substance abuse. Only 5.5 percent experienced a serious mental illness. Data from the National Comorbidity Survey are also used in estimates of the prevalence of mental illness by various government agencies, and are included in the Report on Mental Health by the Surgeon General (U.S. Department of Health and Human Services 1999).

Treatment for those with mental illnesses varies widely, but one important consideration is whether the mental disorder is acute or chronic. Acute conditions and disorders are generally short-term or episodic, and may be triggered by a stressful life event, such as divorce or unemployment, which can lead to a period of depression or other types of mental health problems. Mental health professionals provide various types of therapy that help clients recover more quickly from their illnesses, and also help clients develop coping skills that can help prevent further mental health problems.[3]

Chronic disorders are more constant and long-term (lasting over a year), although individuals will experience recurrent episodes of exacerbated impairment during periods of relative stability. Chronic mental illness causes significant dysfunction in the ability to meet the requirements of daily living. Mechanic (1994) has argued that those with chronic or severe mental illnesses resemble the elderly and disabled in terms of their high need for long-term care and integrated services. Mental health professionals assist clients with their medical needs as well as their social skills, which include activities of daily living, income support, housing, and employment.

The data reported above on the prevalence of mental illness utilize the American Psychological Association's *Diagnostic Statistical Manual of Mental Disorder* to classify mental illness and determine who is mentally ill (American Psychological Association 1994). Yet the existence of mental illness has been subject to a good deal of controversy and debate. One can view mental health and mental illness as residing along a continuum, with varying degrees of illness (or abnormality). Alternatively, mental health and mental illness may represent dichotomous states: one either has a mental illness or one does not.[4] Historically, psychologists have articulated the continuum view of mental health; whereas biomedically oriented researchers and clinicians assume that mental health and illness refer to discrete disease states; that is, one is either mentally ill or one is not. Sociologists tend to favor continuous approaches (Mirowsky and Ross 2002) and Keyes (2002) recently developed and tested a mental health continuum which ranks respondents from languishing (negative mental health) to flourishing (positive mental health).

The psychosocial model of mental illness, dominant until the 1970s, was based upon a continuum definition of mental health. In general terms psychologists focus on the individual factors that affect abnormal thoughts, feelings, and behaviors (Peterson 1999). Psychologists also address interpersonal relationships, childhood socialization, and family strains as important determinants of mental health and illness. Peterson differentiates between four psychological models: the psychoanalytical, cognitive-behavioral, humanistic-existential-phenomenological, and the family systems approach. Each model provides a unique view of human nature and pathology, and offers different approaches to treatment. Rather than emphasizing illness per se, psychologists are often more concerned with optimal states of mental health, and tend to believe that anyone could become ill given the wrong set of circumstances and environmental conditions. Mental health encompasses a number of dimensions, including self-esteem, realization of one's potential, ability to maintain meaningful relationships, psychological well-being, autonomy, and mastery (Ryff 1989). Individuals may seek therapeutic assistance to augment their mental health, rather than merely trying to alleviate symptoms of psychological distress. Psychologists are also likely to emphasize prevention and education to everyone in order to promote conditions of mental health (Grob 1994).

Since the 1980s there has been an increasing emphasis on biological or organic views of mental illness and a corresponding decrease in emphasis on the psychiatric concern with the unconscious, historical development, family dynamics, and social factors (Wilson 1993). From the biomedical perspective mental illness is viewed primarily as a disease of the brain (Horwitz 2002). Included in this approach to mental illness are theories which postulate that mental illness has genetic, biological, biochemical, or neurological causes (Michels and Marzuk 1993). Advances in neuroscience (which combines the findings from several scientific disciplines in order to understand brain structure and human behavior) have vastly increased our understanding of the physiological sources of mental disorder, and have shown that neurological functioning is also influenced by environmental factors.[5] However, the biomedical view tends to emphasize biophysiological factors. Mental illness is defined in terms of deviance from biophysiological norms, and can be diagnosed by the presence of certain symptoms and syndromes.[6] That is, mental illness is a disease with a specific pathology that can be treated (Mishler 1989), primarily with medications which "cure" or "correct" the biological abnormalities.

Sociologists have challenged the biomedical view that mental illnesses merely reflect disease entities (Mirowsky and Ross 1989, 2002; Turner 1987). They focus instead on the social context that affects levels of generalized distress, and on the ways in which certain behaviors are defined as abnormal or deviant.

> The sociological model of illness takes a critical and opposed position on the biochemical model of disease. It treats the concepts of medical science as products of cultural changes . . . the sickness of the patient cannot be understood outside the historical, social, and cultural context of the person (Turner 1987: 9).

Sociologists have not been concerned as much with the etiology of mental illness as with the social processes by which some individuals are labeled mentally ill. Social reaction theory, also referred to as labeling theory, views mental disorder as deviance from institutionalized expectations (Perruci 1974; Scheff 1984; Turner 1987). Mental illness labels involve incomprehensibility (Coulter 1973; Horwitz 1982; Ingleby 1982) since we cannot understand the motives, intentions, and thoughts of the person labeled mentally disordered. Horwitz (1982) argues that the notions of mental illness are rooted in the basic prerequisites of social interaction; that is, we must be able to understand one another. The universal nature of mental illness may stem from the fact that social interaction in all cultures is based upon similar requirements (termed interaction rituals). Rosenberg (1992) argues that mental illness involves role-taking failure: In responding to an individual whom we find to be mentally ill we cannot grasp their perspectives and hence cannot take the role of the other, role-taking failure results. Mental illness is as much an interpersonal phenomenon as it is a biological illness (Doubt 1992); and it represents a failure in interpersonal understanding (Rosenberg 1992: 54).

Horwitz (2002) provides a degree of closure to the debates over the nature of mental illness by differentiating mental diseases (which reflect internal dysfunctions that are found universally) from mental disorders (diseases and disorders in which symptoms are shaped by cultural processes) and from mental illnesses (which reflect labeling processes). He argues that it is critical to differentiate mental disorders from normal reactions to stress (such as depression following divorce) as well as deviance. His critique of diagnostic psychiatry (the classification of mental health problems into DSM categories) points out that only the major psychoses (schizophrenia, bipolar disorder, etc.) meet the criteria of a valid disorder (or a mental disease). For most of the other disorders, the symptoms are not specific indicators of discrete underlying diseases. However, the DSM considers any symptom as evidence of a disorder, regardless of its cause. Hence diagnostic psychiatry overestimates the rates of mental disorder (Horwitz 2002).

The psychosocial, biomedical, and labeling approaches have opposing implications for the treatment of mental illness. Psychologists believe clients need therapy (or professional assistance) in order to help them achieve optimal mental health (whether defined as mentally ill or not). Under the assumptions of the biomedical model (as well as psychologically based theories) a diagnosis of mental illness results in treatment, which is assumed to provide some measure of "cure," or at least alleviate many of its symptoms. Labeling theorists do not deny the potentially positive effects of treatment (Rosenfield 1997), but they argue that labeling produces a stigma that can itself contribute to poor client outcomes (Rosenfield 1997; Link 1987). Many advocates of client empowerment (i.e., see Chamberlain 1979; Estroff 1981) criticize the mental health system for its division of people into "sick" and "well" categories; arguing that in order to become "well," clients must conform to psychiatric definitions of illness and accept the devalued sense of self and self-esteem that results from this acceptance of a stigmatized identity.

Having discussed in very general terms the differences between the psychological, biomedical, and sociological approaches to mental illness, I now examine the providers' views of mental illness and explanations for the causes of mental illness. The consequences of these etiologies for treatment and service delivery will then be considered.

PROVIDER VIEWS OF MENTAL ILLNESS

In in-depth interviews, I asked providers to discuss their earliest conceptions of mental illness, as well as their current theories about its etiology. These responses were examined to determine whether they reflect primarily psychosocial, biomedical, or labeling perspectives on mental illness. I show that the majority of providers combined the three etiologies into a biopsychosocial view. However, before describing providers' etiological assumptions about mental illness, I draw on their descriptions of clients to give the reader a greater sense of how providers view their clients.

Most of the providers found mental illness and their clients "just fascinating":

> I walked on the unit, and we had no idea what to expect, and this bipolar came screaming at the top of her lungs, carrying her breakfast tray trying to catch up with the breakfast man, cigarette dangling out of her mouth, make-up out to here and dangly earrings which didn't match anything, cowboy boots and polyester pants. The other students plastered themselves against the wall to get out of the way. I was just amazed; I fell in love with it right there. (Female nurse case manager in public sector)

As this quote illustrates, most providers had very little previous experience with individuals with either acute or chronic mental illnesses.

> At the beginning I didn't have much experience. Now I love them; they are wonderful people; their values are great; they don't spend their day trying to get what they can get; they are honest, open, loving, caring, supportive of each other. They cut right through the bullshit. (Female MSW case manager in public sector)

This love of and respect for their clients was nearly universal; one provider felt that his clients made "normalcy boring":

> I feel very humble to work with these clients, because I find them to be so courageous. And the quirkiness, and they are just fun. We have one story after another. It makes normalcy boring. (Male MSW case manager in public sector)

In the in-depth interviews I asked providers to describe a critical incident, which gave them insight into both the explicit practices and tacit assumptions of mental health work. Many providers recounted stories about clients who made progress and met some of the initial goals of community integration.

> I'm working with Dawn (a white woman in her 30s); when she first came here she was really frightened of people, now she has some confidence and she'll come and talk with people. Dawn is now thinking on her own, and is even checking into her own transportation. She just wants to be normal, sometimes there such a stigma that they are less than because they go to the mental health center. (Female MSW case manager in public sector)

Many providers were particularly proud of making progress with a recalcitrant client.

> I have an older client, a man, who was a welder, had a drinking and substance abuse problem, but was "normal." He had a breakdown, went to the hospital and was diagnosed as schizophrenic; subsequently he had 45 different hospitalizations. He's been on my caseload for 2 years now, another case manager found him too difficult and violent—but I like to work with difficult clients. Since I've worked with him, he's only been in the hospital once, he's in day treatment, I got him an apartment, and he's only been evicted once for letting a lot of other people into his house, he no longer uses coke, and he only drinks occasionally. (Male MSW case manager in public sector)

While half of the providers related clients' success stories, the other half related stories of clients who failed, who needed a great deal of help, or who faced insurmountable problems.

I'll use a client who was diagnosed with schizophrenia, who doesn't really believe he has a mental illness, and refuses medication because he sees them as poison, and now and then his symptoms can become quite strong . . . and he's inundated with spaceships, and things that come out of the sky, and he tries to maintain himself. While he's trying to maintain—he isolates himself, he doesn't trust himself out in public, and his only contact is once a week when I come to talk to him. And we talk about that (i.e., the illness), concentrating on trees and nature, and limiting the stimuli in his environment. We gradually ride out the symptoms, and then we start focusing on paying bills, and umm, getting groceries, and keeping an apartment. (Male MSW case manager in public sector)

Often the problems were not unique to individuals diagnosed with a mental illness.

I have a client whose boyfriend was beating her up and throwing her down the stairs. I wanted her to take out a warrant, but she didn't want to do that, so I got her into the battered woman's shelter yesterday. Today we had to go get her clothes, so I called the police from the convenience store near her apartment. When we got there the boyfriend was there and he was livid. I worry more about the environment than my client; mentally ill clients, after you work with them for awhile, are much more predictable than other folks. You can tell when they are starting to have problems, but with other people you can't tell what they will do. (Male case manager in public sector)

The hardest clients "to shake" were those who had died, or who had committed suicide. One provider recounted stories about accidental deaths: one client left the stove gas on, another committed suicide, and a third died in an emergency, "So we had three deaths [on a team] in three months, and that was hard." Another provider told of having to pack up the personal belongings of one of his clients after her suicide. Often, violence was a typical feature of client's lives.

I had one client laying around in the driveway, walking around in his underwear. I went out there when I was called in by the cops; I made him an appointment as I realized he needed help. A week later he was dead; he'd been shot, broke into somebody's house and helped himself to food and beer and the owner shot him dead. I have another client, someone with AIDS, and ex-IV user, prostitute, arrested six times last year for prostitution. Arrested twice so far this year, only a month apart. Well, she went out and got herself picked up by two guys and was almost killed. They beat her to within an hour of her life; she'd been hit with a tire iron on the skull, it split her ear. I just don't know what to do with her. (Male case manager in public sector)

Knowing how to help a client depends on the provider's views about the origins of mental illness. Providers adhering to a primarily psychosocial view of mental illness emphasize personality, socialization, and family factors as critical to their understanding of mental health and illness. Very few of the providers who worked primarily with clients with severe mental illnesses adhered to purely a psychosocial view of mental illness, though a few private clinicians viewed mental health problems in this manner. One's beliefs about mental illness have an important experiential basis; providers in the public sector work almost exclusively with clients with chronic mental illnesses, whereas providers in the private sector work exclusively with those with more acute mental health problems.

Providers with their own practices were able to select the types of clients they worked with and, in fact, most of them specialized in one type of client population or mental health problem, such as couples therapy, family therapy, depression, substance abuse, homosexuality, or sexual abuse. None of the private clinicians worked with many clients with severe, persistent mental illness. One reported, "My whole caseload is 'worried well' except some of the sexual abuse survivors." Providers in private practice tended to articulate views of mental health and illness that were consistent with the psychological approach appropriate to their current practice, whether it was psychoanalytical, cognitive-behavioral, humanistic-existential, or family systems. Many of these providers emphasized psychosocial factors in describing the sources of mental health problems.

> I help them to find that seed that is themselves on the inside, and really develop that self, and shed the things that have not been helpful, that they learned in their years of experience . . . I just think we get a lot of wounds. (Female MSW in private practice)

Another private clinician articulated the classical psychoanalytical view of mental illness: "Unless you make the unconscious conscious, you can't deal with all the urges and drives."

However, when asked to discuss serious, or chronic, mental illnesses, the private providers (many of whom had previous work experience with this population in the public sector) emphasized biological mechanisms as well as psychosocial factors.

> I think mental illness is the same way (as addiction); we are born with a genetic disposition toward addiction or depression, depending on what our circumstances are like; the stress, the trauma, it will clearly impact on the severity and degree of the mental health problem. (Female MSW in private practice)

A few of the providers in the public sector identified with a "pure" psychosocial view of mental illness, and they qualified their understanding by noting that their views had changed since working with individuals with chronic mental health conditions. One provider in the public sector offered a view of mental illness that was clearly in accord with the psychosocial approach dominant until the 1970s: "We all strive for emotional health, some just fall short." Yet this male MSW case manager continued:

> It is a brain disease that impacts on the social, physical, and interpersonal levels. These people didn't get this way by being confused. How much stress in early life has to do with it is anybody's guess, just like cardiovascular disease, but I think of it as primarily a bio-chemical problem.

The vast majority of providers combined elements of the psychosocial approach with a biomedical view of mental illness as a disease. This was almost universally true of providers with advanced degrees, as well as those with nursing degrees.

> I believe it's organic, certainly it's a combination of environment and organic, but organic is there. And medication is necessary for that. I got that from [graduating college], you can tell I'm a nurse. It's organic; mental illness is a disease. (Female nurse in public sector)

Another MSW case worker argued that

> It's definitely caused by chemical imbalances in the brain, and that's significantly affected by peoples' families, their lives, abuse. And that daily living stress affects someone with a chemical imbalance even more.

Some providers viewed biology as primary, though psychosocial and environmental factors were also important triggers: "There's definitely a biological component to it. I think there is something other than that, that can trigger that biological problem."

> My personal feeling is that probably a lot of it is genetic. External influences such as drug abuse and that sort of thing can make what would be minimal symptoms much worse. An awful lot of it has to do with genetic makeup and chemical imbalances. (Male case manager in public sector)

Other providers viewed environmental forces as primary, but felt that biological disposition had to be present.

> Back when I got out (of school) there was a big division over whether it was learned or genetic—I believe you have a strong genetic disposition, but the environment will make the difference—push you over the edge, or nurture and protect you. (Female case manager in public sector)

Given their belief in the biomedical basis for mental illness, most providers felt medication was appropriate and necessary: "I'm a believer in medications; I equate mental illness with a physical illness." Another provider stated more flatly, "Meds are the main thing, the other stuff is around the edges."

In my earlier research on outpatient commitment (conducted in the early 1980s) I found that providers medicalized the illness of their patients and they felt that medication was the "bottom line" of treatment (Scheid-Cook 1991; Scheid-Cook 1992). "Medication is what helps most of them deal with their mental illness and to stabilize, not therapy or talking over their problems." In this earlier research I also had access to client's medical records, and found that while the majority were receiving medication, very few received any alternative treatments, psychosocial therapy, or skills training (Scheid-Cook 1991). However, the data reflect the gaps in community-based services prevalent in the 1980s (Grob 1994) rather than provider's preferred mode of treatment.

Only a few providers I interviewed were critical of the biomedical model; they felt those with mental illness were no different: "They have limitations, just like everyone." One provider referred to clients with mental illness as "people in pain, it's not just a diagnosis."

> They have a disability, but lots of people have a disability; either they never had the chance to learn certain skills because of the disability, or they lost them because of the psychiatric problems—maybe they ended up in the hospital, god only knows what happened to them. A lot of it is that every person has a different level of what they can and can't control. (Female nurse case manager in public sector)

These providers were critical of what they perceived as an over-reliance on psychiatric medication.

> I really had no early conception of mental illness. I now know they are individuals the same as I am, and I'm kind of angry at our system for how they were treated—just given meds, not taught any skills. (Female MSW case manager)

Providers believe that rather than medication, skills training or various forms of psychosocial therapy are necessary to deal with the problems in daily living caused by mental illness. The majority of those interviewed did not believe that medication was effective as the sole means of treatment. Instead, they agreed with Engel's (1980) delineation of the biopsychosocial model; clients need a combination of medication (biological), therapy (psychological), and skills training (social). This model has been prevalent in the mental health field, and was reinforced by the development of Community Support Programs (CSP) and Assertive Community Treatment (ACT) in the 1980s.

BIOPSYCHOSOCIAL REHABILITATION AND
CLINICAL MANAGEMENT

The biopsychosocial model integrates biological mechanisms, psychological processes, and social influences on mental abnormality, and is widely accepted by psychologists (Peterson 1999). An integrated etiology was the predominant view of serious mental illness held by providers I interviewed (especially those in the public sector). Providers in private practice worked primarily with the "worried well" whereas those in the public sector worked primarily with clients with severe, persistent mental illnesses. Consequently, providers in private practice were more likely to view themselves as "clinicians" who provide therapy. Providers in the public sector were case managers, who performed a brokerage role. The views and beliefs about mental health and illness held by professional groups is an important institutional demand, which will shape the delivery of mental health services and consequently the work of mental health care providers. In this section I will look more closely at the development and implications of the biopsychosocial model of treatment.

Biopsychosocial rehabilitation focuses on the consequences, rather than the causes, of mental illness. Medication is still primary, because it is the only technology available which deals with the overt manifestations of the illness. Psychosocial rehabilitation also deals with the stigma, lowered self-esteem, and loss of community support that result from the mental illness. In addition to medication, clients are assigned to a case manager, and offered a variety of other mental health programs to meet their needs, for example, partial hospitalization, vocational clubhouses, skills training, or occupational therapy. A case manager works with the client to coordinate the diverse services needed to live in the community. Consequently, the case manager spends time with the client out in the community, making sure that they have housing and that they are able to manage daily life.[7] Much time is spent dealing with other social service agencies, such as departments of social services, criminal justice agencies, vocational rehabilitation, nursing homes, halfway houses, inpatient units, and other health care providers. Providers also negotiate with their clients' families, landlords, and employers, to ensure they are receiving adequate social support in the community. In addition, the provider may also be responsible for their clients' medication compliance. Providers are also expected to combat stigma by engaging in community outreach and education. However, most providers would still like the opportunity to use therapeutic skills, and many of those I interviewed criticized biopsychosocial rehabilitation for its overemphasis on management.

> A lot of these folks need therapy, not just managing. But if they have just a case manager, they get managing, not therapy. Once they start working with

a case manager the case manager just manages, makes sure they get meds, housing, health care needs are met. Its not therapy. But I think therapy does help with mental illness. (Male MA case manager in public sector)

Other providers felt that there was too much emphasis on medication, and that more therapy was needed.

Personally I don't think they need as much medication; some do need medication, but they need to be able to discuss their problems and have someone explain what is happening; they [i.e., case managers] need to take more time to speak to the patients. (Female case manager in public sector).

These providers believe that not all of their clients' needs are met with biopsychosocial rehabilitation, and know that medication has displaced more traditional forms of therapy. Consequently, the provider becomes little more than a manager who oversees treatment largely provided by others. They no longer engage in therapy on their own. Providers experience a reduced sense of professional and personal accomplishment when their clinical role is reduced to that of coordinator rather than provider of care. The relationship with clients has been curtailed by a model that at first glance appears very broad, but that may in fact limit the kinds of relationships providers are able to establish with their clients.

Another source of ideological conflict within the parameters of biopsychosocial rehabilitation is that of normalization versus empowerment. In working with clients with chronic mental illnesses, case management is oriented toward "normalization"; the goal is that clients will resume normal lives in the community. The concept of normalization originated in Europe and was popularized in America by Wolfensberger (Greenspan and Cerreto 1989). Normalization is realized through the application of various techniques that result in behaviors characterized as culturally normative. Medication, skills training, and vocational preparation are all viewed as essential to the process of normalization.

While on the surface normalization would seem to be a worthwhile service goal, in fact it has been criticized for its focus on conformity, and for its assumption that the culturally normative values of the wider society are worth aspiring to (Anderton et al. 1989; Hattersley 1991). Bayley (1991: 88) has suggested that conformity to Western ideals of individualistic achievement and independence may be "profoundly unhelpful" to those with mental disabilities. Lefley (1984) argues that such emphasis on Western ideals represents a type of professional ethnocentrism that may be inappropriate to clients in different cultural contexts as well as minorities. Normalization efforts in rehabilitation contribute to the social control functions of negative labeling because an individual is expected to *adjust* to society (Susman 1994) and must therefore internalize the socially devalued identity that has been ascribed to them. Consequently, an emphasis upon normalization may result in lower self-esteem (as described above). Further-more, normalization may also work against self-acceptance and conscious-ness-raising (Szivos and Travers 1988), processes that are critical to client empowerment.

Empowerment is an alternative to the traditional notion of mental health that is based on the advocacy model was first presented by Rose and Black (1985). While an extension of consumer rights was part of the origi-nal ideology of the community care movement, empowerment explicitly rejects the idea of professional intervention, whether from a psychosocial or a biomedical framework (Paulson 1992). Instead, clients are "empow-ered" to obtain the resources that will give them increased control over their environments (Hasenfeld and Chesler 1989), and that will further client autonomy in the community as well as self-esteem. As one provider said, "You don't have self-esteem if you are not empowered to take charge of your life." As agents, clients (or consumers) initiate service intervention and are authorized to assume control over the direction of their treatment and ultimately, their life. McLean (2000) provides an overview of the evo-lution of the consumer movement, noting how the concept of empower-ment has evolved from independence *from* the system, to the exercise of choice *within* the system (2000: 837). The consumer movement has also spawned a number of self-help alternatives to traditional mental health care. Yet McLean notes that both traditional and consumer alternatives are being curtailed by the cost-saving logics of managed care.

Within an empowerment framework, providers do not merely coordi-nate care, they advocate for consumers and help them formulate their con-cerns into specific strategies for action (Paulson 1992). A provider might advocate for the consumers' right to refuse medication and to live in set-tings of their own choice, whether floridly symptomatic or not. Case man-agers would also work with consumers to develop workplace alternatives where mental illness was more widely accepted, and "individuals are ac-cepted for their quirkiness."

Neugeboren (1999) describes a number of programs that are based on the ideal of empowerment and which seek to move clients to recovery. Re-covery is a recent outgrowth of the consumer movement and has become a guiding principal to mental health care reform (U.S. Department of Health and Human Services 1997). Wisconsin has organized its mental health care system around the ideal of recovery (Blue Ribbon Commission on Mental Health Care 1997). Recovery is described by Jacobson and Greenley (2001) as including internal conditions (hope, healing, empow-erment, and connection) and external conditions (human rights, positive culture of healing, services to link clients to the community). Recovery en-compasses both normalization and empowerment and advocates col-laborative consumer/provider relationships. Markowitz (2001) finds that recovery-based treatment programs (which provided social and vocational skills) had the effect of increasing a client's self-esteem and sense of mastery, which then resulted in decreased symptomatology. Markowitz (2001) also raises concerns that managed care will limit the nonclinical services central to recovery. Neugeboren (1999) raises the same concerns and argues that once clients are stabilized on medications, their need for social services increases.

COMMUNITY-BASED CARE

The ascendancy of the biopsychosocial model was concurrent with the development of community-based care for those with chronic mental illness. As noted earlier, community-based care relies on a social, rather than a medical, model of mental illness. Minkoff (1997: 15) summarizes the broad institutional demands placed upon CMHCs, which he refers to as the original community mental health ideology:

1. CMHCs should address the needs of the whole community as defined by the catchment area.
2. CMHC services should be available to everyone.
3. Mental health services should be provided by organized systems that are responsive to the communities they serve.
4. CMHCs should emphasize crisis intervention and reliance on natural support systems that promote normalization and community integration.
5. CMHCs should emphasize the provision of community-based alternatives.

People with chronic mental illnesses need supportive services in order to live in the community (i.e., income support, housing, vocational rehabilitation, skills training). Part of the early failure of deinstitutionalization was the inability of community mental health providers to provide or coordinate the necessary support services (Ahmed and Plog 1976; Mechanic and Rochefort 1990; Morrissey et al. 1980; Rochefort 1989; Shadish et al. 1989). Rather than therapy, these clients needed supportive services and case management (Mechanic 1986).

Case management coordinates the necessary services and supports needed to maintain the client in the community (Dill 2001). It became the primary mode of treatment for individuals with chronic mental illness by the mid-1980s (Harris and Bergman 1987), and mental health providers had to become case managers rather than therapists. At first providers resisted this redefinition of their role, in part because case management was viewed as not challenging or rewarding professionally (see Deitchman 1980 for a concise and humorous critique of case management). Rubin and

Johnson (1984) found that MSW students had little interest or preference for work with the chronically mentally ill, or for case-management services in general. At CARE the movement to case management involved conflict over the new job title, and a compromise was reached with the designation of case managers as psychosocial rehabilitation counselors. This title allowed providers at CARE to retain some identification with their older therapeutic role (i.e., counselor), while incorporating the new case-management role (i.e., psychosocial rehabilitation).

The debate over case management no doubt reflected professional conflict between providers with clinical backgrounds who emphasized the cure of illnesses versus those with rehabilitation practitioners focused on helping the clients adjust to their illnesses. Clinical providers focus on symptoms, whereas rehabilitation focuses upon improving levels of functioning. Clinically oriented practitioners tend to assume a positive correlation between symptomatology and other client outcomes, whereas rehabilitation practitioners do not. This debate has been partially resolved by the integration of clinical and psychosocial outcomes in many treatment programs and assessment instruments (for example, the Global Assessment Scale).

Besides professional beliefs and values, governmental policies also have an impact on the availability of services (that is, they are another important institutional demand). In order to correct the initial failures of community-based health care, the National Institute of Mental Health (NIMH) provided funding for training programs and services research (Grob 1994). One of the most critical programs supported by the NIMH was the Community Support Program (CSP), an organization developed to meet the needs of those with chronic mental illness in the community. As detailed by Tessler and Goldman (1982) CSPs provide coordinated case management, assessment, identification, and diagnosis of those in need of crisis intervention (to prevent hospitalization), psychiatric treatment, support for activities of daily living, psychosocial rehabilitation, client advocacy, and the provision (or coordination) of residential, vocational, and recreational services. Clearly, CSPs were based upon a biopsychosocial view of mental illness.

Many states mandated that community mental health centers meet the standards of CSP certification, which often required that case managers meet certain professional criteria (an advanced degree or certification in psychosocial rehabilitation).[8] Consequently, case management became professionally legitimated, and many mental health care providers now receive extensive professional socialization in biopsychosocial rehabilitation. Yet case management may well represent a curtailment of the clinical role as workers become managers but not providers of care. Many providers receive initial professional training in counseling and are primarily motivated by the ideal of establishing an emotional bond with their clients. The tension providers experience between management and care is significant for understanding the difficulties posed by managed care. Providers become the entities who are managed, and their care-giving labor is limited by criteria of scientific efficacy. This study shows that managed care reifies the view of mental illness as a disease entity and promotes a view of treatment as a technical procedure that produces predictable client level outcomes; supportive services may be deemphasized if they are not deemed cost-effective or clinically efficacious. Such a view of treatment further restricts the emotional labor of the mental health care provider, and places this labor under increased bureaucratic control. The next chapter provides a more general introduction to the concept of treatment ideology, and describes the treatment ideologies that prevailed prior to the ascendancy of managed care.

NOTES

1. The recipients of mental health services were referred to as "patients" when the primary mode of care was inpatient hospitalization and medication, "clients" with the development of community-based services, and "consumers" with the advent of client empowerment. Some advocates use the term "survivor" to refer to the idea that individuals "survive" the mental health system. Since I am not sure I believe individuals with severe mental illnesses always have the degree of choice implied by the term consumer, I will use the term client because it has the advantage of focusing on the provider/client relationship and also applies to individuals who receive services in both public as well as private care settings.

2. State mental hospitals have not disappeared; in fact, most of the several hundred state mental hospitals created since 1773 are still in existence (in 1990 the National Institute of Mental Health listed 286). Furthermore, in the mid-1990s the average state still spent 57 percent of their mental health dollars on hospitals (Dowdall 1996). While patient populations are sharply reduced, state hospitals still provide custodial care to those who cannot survive in the community. Yet most state hospitals can no longer be characterized as warehouses—they have diversified and now provide a broad range of outpatient and rehabilitation services to assorted patient populations (Gudeman 1988).

3. Some mental health professionals are able to work with their clients to achieve optimal mental health and emphasize increased insight and self awareness. This is especially true of providers in private practice who are able to work with clients who can afford ongoing therapy on a fee-for-service basis.

4. Some scholars (Coulter 1979; Foucault 1975; Szasz 1963, 1984) argue that mental illness is a construct that refers to actions viewed as deviant, and therefore in need of social control.

5. Some psychiatrists advance a view of the social brain, demonstrating that the brain in fact responds to the environment. For example, Eisenberg (1995: 1563) argues that "the human brain is socially constructed . . . the cytoarchitectonics of the cerebral cortex are sculpted by input from the social environment because socialization shapes the essential human attributes of our species."

6. There has been a great deal of academic debate over whether mental illnesses can be diagnosed and classified (i.e., psychiatric nomenclature). Mirowsky and Ross (1989) have argued the psychiatric diagnoses are reified measurements, that what is assessed by diagnostic frameworks such as the DSM are psychiatrists' views of mental illness. Their argument has received empirical support by those who have studied the processes by which different types of behaviors come to be defined as mental illnesses (Caplan 1995; Kirk and Kutchins 1992).

7. Dill (2001) argues that case management is an individualized solution to the problem of system integration.

8. For example Wisconsin required that each mental health catchment area provide a CSP by 1984. In many counties, the CSP provided services to those with primarily chronic mental illnesses while the traditional community mental health center focused on the needs of other client populations.

3   Ideologies of Care
Parent, Caretaker, Advocate, Best Friend

Ideology is an abstract system of ideas mediated by operational philosophies. Operational philosophies are systems of ideas and procedures for implementing therapeutic ideologies under specific institutional conditions.
(Strauss et al. 1964: 360)

As Strauss et al. (1964: 361) first articulated, beliefs about care make a difference in the treatment provided and in the structure of organizational
roles; ideology is critical to understanding "what is done for patients and
who does what kind of work." An analysis of providers' treatment ideologies is also critical to understanding their emotional labor, because it is
treatment ideology that identifies the operative feeling rules necessary for
performance of the clinical role. Ideologies also help providers reconcile
conflicting institutional demands. I begin with a general theoretical discussion of the nature and importance of treatment ideologies and then examine where treatment ideologies are acquired and the different sources
of beliefs about mental health work. Treatment ideologies encompass the
feeling rules that direct clinical work and specify the appropriate role providers "play" as well as their ideal goals of treatment. Treatment ideologies are also central to the work identity of providers.

Treatment ideologies bind people together. Consequently, different ideologies can be a source of conflict between professional groups. Jurisdictional disputes (see Abbott 1988) revolve around questions of who has the
power to decide which model of care a given group or organization ought
to pursue. In the second half of the chapter I look at the specific treatment
ideologies exhibited by the providers I interviewed, and examine the
prevalence of diverse treatment ideologies in the two public sector organizations I studied in depth. The primary source of data is the qualitative,
in-depth interviews in which providers discuss their treatment practices.
While I use some information obtained from private clinicians, I focus on
the treatment ideologies of those in the public sector who work with clients

with severe, persistent illnesses. Not only do these providers work with similar clients, they also face similar institutional and organizational constraints, and these have a bearing on treatment ideologies and practices.

AN EXPLANATION OF TREATMENT IDEOLOGY

I define treatment ideology as the complex set of beliefs health care providers hold about mental health, illness, and treatment (see Scheid 1994 for my first definition of treatment ideology). These beliefs consist of specific theories about the etiology (cause) of mental illness, the role of the patient, and the validity of various treatments (many of which were discussed in the previous chapter). This definition of treatment ideology is analogous to that of psychiatric ideology developed by Strauss et al. (1964) in their classic study of psychiatric patients. Strauss et al. (ibid.: 8) define a psychiatric ideology as "shared or collective sets of psychiatric ideas" about the etiology and treatment of mental illness.[1] Taking this definition a little further, Eaton et. al (1990) define medical ideology as sets of ideas related to diagnoses that have action consequences. That is, medical ideologies guide the treatment decisions and behaviors of practitioners. They tell the provider what to do and how to do it. Luhrmann (2000) provides an excellent account of the treatment ideologies of psychiatric residents. Ideology, which contains both "is" and "ought" properties, "is a set of ideas with affective overtones that describe both the world that is, and the world that ought to be" (Wilson 1992: 19). In a discussion of how medical professionals do their work, Abbott (1992) also focuses on diagnosis and treatment as central to constructions of appropriate actions. Thus, treatment ideologies are organized around views about mental health and illness.

However, it is important to bear in mind that treatment ideologies are not an individual's beliefs or opinions. Rather, they are the property of a collectivity or organization (see Berger and Luckmann 1967), and serve the important function of legitimating existing ways of doing things and structural arrangements. Ideologies are the outcomes of complex processes of intersubjective negotiation between individuals (Fine 1984), and cannot be reduced to individual beliefs or actions. These negotiations generally occur within organizational frameworks (Levitt and March 1988). The fact that ideologies are collective in nature does not imply that ideological beliefs are not held by individuals. Negotiations between individuals produce organizational classifications and typifications.

> Ideology is both personal and shared. Simultaneously it is a property of the social actor; it is enacted in a relationship, and is a property of the group or community. . . . In its cognitive and emotive components we see the importance of the actor; in its enactment we see the role of the community, class, or social network. (Fine and Sandstrom 1993: 32)

The collective site of treatment ideologies is the organization where providers meet, learn, and work. Ideology is an important reference for action; ideologies can guide and channel the specific behaviors and performances of providers as well as have a direct impact on the formal structure of the organization. Consequently, ideologies overlap both conceptually and empirically with aspects of the organization's culture (Goll and Zeitz 1991). Ideologies bind people together via common beliefs (i.e., culture), and help them enact their roles within the organization (Trice and Beyer 1993). There is a good bit of literature describing how human service workers and organizations produce the relevant characteristics of their clients, which then legitimate a particular response to these clients (Cicourel 1968; Holstein 1992; Pfohl 1978; Salaman 1980). That is, organizations do not merely *process* people, they produce them as well (Holstein 1992; Salaman 1980).

While ideologies are central features of an organization's culture, they can arise from past experiences and interpretations, prior socialization, training, and concrete work experiences. This is especially true of the treatment ideologies that guide clinical work. Professionals come to a given job or organization with a set of treatment ideologies developed through their training and previous occupational experience. The current organization then plays an important role in shaping, or solidifying, previously held beliefs. In this manner, treatment ideologies are reproduced, and may also be an important source of organizational change.

Imagine it is 1986 and a young clinician, fresh from graduate school and clinical rotation at the University of Madison-Wisconsin, where the model for Assertive Community Treatment (ACT) was developed, has joined the staff at a small rural community mental health center in the South, where the primary form of treatment had been inpatient hospitalization and medication. This clinician might be able to introduce the mental health organization to a new treatment ideology, for example, a new way of dealing with chronically mental ill clients in the community. Or the mental health center and its staff may be too set in its ways (organizational inertia), and may resist efforts to change or innovate. The views of the young clinician may be viewed as "utopian" and completely unworkable. Karl Mannheim (1936) distinguished ideologies (which support the status quo) from utopias (which challenge the status quo). Ideologies not only protect established beliefs and practices (legitimation), they can also provide a shield from the "constant threat of discrepancies arising from individual (or sectional) perceptions, or from new 'external' developments" (Thompson 1980: 229).

In practical terms, young clinicians (such as the one in my example) will probably have to conform to dominant organizational ideologies and practices because they have little power and little choice (Martin 1992). The organization is not likely to make a risky change to its practices, unless the "new practices are emotionally laden and ideologically appealing" (D'Aunno et al. 1991: 658) or yield some tangible benefit. As will be shown in discussions of managed care in later chapters, financial benefits have had quite an impact on the treatment practices of clinicians in private practice.

My example of the young clinician raises the question of the relationship between the individual and the organization: which is the primary source of treatment ideology? Two alternative theories explain the source of organizational beliefs and practices (Findlay et al. 1990). The *importation hypothesis* stipulates that organizational practices result from pre-existing attitudes and behaviors of participants. These practices may originate in professional beliefs about appropriate treatment which are held by groups external to the organization (professional beliefs are an important institutional constraint to which organizations are expected to conform). The alternative to the importation hypothesis is the *homogenization hypothesis*, which argues that participants are largely shaped by the organization. Critical to this hypothesis is the notion of relative power of the organization, and the power held by professionals who work within the organization, the source of many studies of bureaucratic and professional conflict. Organizations attempt to select employees whose perspectives fit within the overall mission of the organization and individuals also seek employment in organizations that appear "like-minded," although of course such choice is constrained by many different factors, such as availability of jobs and the individual's mobility. One of the critical concerns today is whether managed mental health care will limit the power and autonomy of mental health professionals by imposing organizational constraints on treatment. We will look more closely at this issue in the following chapters.

It is also necessary to examine the source of a given belief system and the relative power and status of the group that promotes it. The external environment plays an important role in shaping both organizational ideologies and individual beliefs. The institutional environment (DiMaggio and Powell 1991; Meyer and Scott 1983; Zucker 1987) consists of the normative beliefs and societal preferences for the treatment of mental illness. A concrete example of the effect of the institutional environment is the societal preference for community-based treatment as opposed to custodial care for individuals with mental illness. Popular books such as Goffman's *Asylums* and Kesey's *One Flew Over the Cuckoo's Nest* helped propel deinstitutionalization and the closing of large state asylums in the 1970s (though other factors, such as fiscal reform and the development of psychotropic drugs were also critical). In order to maintain legitimacy and ultimately to secure resources from the external environment, mental health care organizations must conform to institutional expectations about appropriate mental health care. For example, Ziegenfuss (1983) examined organizational congruence with new environmental pressures that emphasized patient's rights. In the 1970s it was difficult to offer mentally ill people anything more than hospitalization, while currently, it is very difficult to commit an individual to a hospital.

In addition to broad societal normative beliefs, professional norms and practices also constitute an important source of treatment ideology. Hasenfeld (1992) has referred to the beliefs that justify services offered to clients by providers as practice ideologies; obviously, practice and treatment ideologies are analogous concepts. Professional and community standards may converge, diverge, or there may be a lag between the two. There is also likely to be conflict between different professional groups working with the same type of clients or in the same organization. Mental health care providers come from diverse professional backgrounds: psychiatry, psychology, social work, and nursing being the most common fields. Because definitions of mental illness and effective treatment are ambiguous (Mechanic 1986) different professional groups often hold contradictory ideologies. Meyerson (1991) found that social workers in hospital settings experienced contradictions between medical and psychosocial practices, and between detachment and involvement with clients. Given the diverse sources of treatment ideologies in a given organization, there may well be a "multiplicity of ideologies" that are not "necessarily logically consistent" (Trice and Beyer 1993: 37). Consequently, Hasenfeld (1986: 14) has described mental health organizations as "rich in ideologies and poor in effective technologies." Psychiatrists and nurses may be more likely to emphasize a biomedical view of mental illness, social workers may accept rehabilitation, and counselors and psychologists may believe psychotherapy is the most effective way to deal with mental illness. Furthermore, as Meyerson (1991) found, contradictory beliefs can be held by individuals of the same profession.

Within the psychiatric and social work literatures, theories about the treatment of mental illness are numerous and reflect different schools of thought about the etiology of mental illness. These theories result in competing counseling models. The concept of a model is more restrictive than that of a treatment ideology and refers to specific procedures or approaches that need not be legitimated by the organization or others with whom one works. MacDonald (1991) describes eighteen counseling models in mental health. The larger number of models correspond to existing treatment approaches described in textbooks on psychotherapy or mental health care, and vary from profession to profession. As Benner (1984) has shown with respect to nurses, theoretical belief systems are modified by practical work experiences. In the mental health field a therapist may prefer existential humanism, but may find that this approach does not work well with individuals with chronic mental illnesses and problems with living. It is important to keep in mind that models can be held by individuals and need not be affirmed by coworkers while treatment ideologies are a collective property. Treatment ideologies (as opposed to models or beliefs) consist of a *set* of beliefs linking evaluations with behavior (Fine and Sandstrom 1993) and hence have consequences for the prevailing organizational structure.

The literature on treatment practices relies upon constructs based upon established models of care, and does not adequately explore the beliefs about the etiology of illness and treatment underlying these models. An exception is MacDonald (1991), who describes the philosophical orientations that underpin the eighteen models of treatment. These philosophies are based upon different domain assumptions about the source of mental illness (the individual or the social environment) and the individual responsible for subsequent changes in the client (self or others).[2] These assumptions about etiology and treatment determine specific treatment ideologies. Heaney and Burke (1995) use data collected from employees at group homes to argue that normalization as a pervasive ideology of care is the guiding ideology for community residential care.

To summarize the discussion thus far, treatment ideologies are shaped by cultural, social, professional, and organizational contexts. Treatment ideologies shape treatment decisions and practices and specify the feeling rules to which providers will attempt to adhere. Consequently treatment ideologies direct the emotional labor of providers and influence the care received by the client. I now turn to the empirical description of the treatment ideologies held by the providers I have interviewed in-depth.

TREATMENT IDEOLOGY: SPECIFICATION
OF ROLES AND GOALS

In earlier work I developed a typology of treatment ideologies (Scheid 1994) from in-depth interviews with providers, as well as from the literature on mental health treatment. The typology is based upon two axes, which represent the domain assumptions about two fundamental questions. The first question concerns the appropriate role for the provider. That is, how does the provider behave toward the client? A given role specifies the feeling rules and attitude a provider will assume with their client. Will the provider act as a parent or a friend? A caretaker or an advocate? The second question concerns the goal of treatment. What does the provider work toward? What constitutes success? A provider's treatment role, as well as the goal of treatment, will vary from client to client. However, since the providers I interviewed worked primarily with clients with severe, persistent mental illnesses, some commonality in terms of treatment ideology is to be expected.

There are three possible roles that the mental health provider can take: custodial, supportive, or facilitative. Many providers working in inpatient organizations or institutionalized settings (Goffman 1961) would describe their role as primarily custodial (though they may not fully embrace this role). The primary function of a custodial role is to meet the client's basic needs and to maintain a sense of order in the institutional environment. A custodial role can also be found in outpatient settings; many providers working in partial hospitalization or clubhouses find themselves playing a custodial role, and treat their clients as young children in need of constant supervision and care. Often such care consists of regulating the clients' behavior.

> I am in the role of being the heavy, like no—you have to take your meds in front of us. I'm sorry if they make you tired, if you don't do it I'm going to call your probation office. (Male rehabilitation counselor in a supported employment program)

Providers may also see their role as primarily supportive; they provide ongoing assistance to their clients. Supportive providers help the clients meet their basic social needs, such as finding a job or a place to live. They may help the clients shop for groceries or perform routine housekeeping chores. Often support consists of merely listening, or being there when the clients need someone. The provider's supportive role is central to the case management model, and emphasizes brokerage (or management) functions.

> We are the mediators. We do the really hard work. We spend time with these folks, we're the ones that have to negotiate what these people really need, like an apartment. It takes an enormous amount of energy. (Female MSW case manager)

Finally, providers may see their role as facilitating or enabling the clients to meet their treatment goals. Here the client is responsible for achieving a measure of success, but the providers facilitate that process in whatever way they can. Facilitative roles were predominant among providers in private practice; over two-thirds used the word "facilitator" to describe their role. One provider in practice defined this facilitative role as one who is a "motivator to look at options in life and then support the process." Another saw herself as a "cheerleader—I get them to go even when they are too depressed to get themselves out of bed." However, the facilitator role is also common among providers in the public sector.

The second dimension along which treatment ideologies can be arrayed is the appropriate goal of treatment. There are three possible goals: control, adjustment, or autonomy. Treatment may be oriented toward control of the client, such as involuntary commitment, use of restraints, or use of medications to tranquilize a client. Generally the goal of such treatment is to prevent the client from being "a nuisance to the community" or to "help them to stay out of trouble with the law" or, more seriously, to keep them from harming themselves or others.

More often the intended outcome of treatment is to adjust the client to the social world of the mental health organization or the larger community.

Providers want their clients to achieve stability in the community, to conform to wider expectations, or to at least appear normal. The term "stabilization" was used by a majority of providers in public practice when asked to describe their treatment goals. They used this term to mean keeping the client "out of the hospital, stabilized on medications, able to function in a more independent living environment, and to have more effective social interactions."

The third treatment goal is autonomy. Providers want clients to gain increasing control over their lives and thus have greater opportunities for independent choice. Rather than maintaining the clients, the provider prefers that clients no longer need mental health care, or that they will be "able to live in a place of their own choice and [be] comfortable with the mental and physical resources" available to him or her. Often this means that clients will have some tolerance of, or insight into, their illnesses as a means of controlling the illness and their lives. Once again, providers in private practice were more likely to stress autonomy as the goal of treatment, and they generally said that only the client could determine the appropriate goal of treatment. As one provider said, "It depends on the goal of the client."

Both dimensions can be seen as stages in a continuum of treatments, and a given provider can serve different roles with different clients, or may assume these different roles with the same client. Clients may begin their treatment career needing to be controlled; hence the providers must play a custodial role. The clients may then "progress" to the point where they are working toward greater community adjustment, and the providers begin to play a supportive role. Finally, the client may move to a stage at which they can assume greater autonomy, and then the providers may become facilitators, or advisors, no longer providing support, but offering a different type of guidance. However, while the goal of treatment may change with each client, or as a given client makes "progress," providers likely feel most comfortable in one type of role regardless of the treatment goal. Facilitators are not likely to enjoy having to pay a more supportive or custodial role, and a supportive provider may lack the skills to become a facilitator. While social roles are acquired via social interaction, a provider's personal inclination makes some roles difficult to assume, raising the question of the relationship of emotional labor and identity. This question will be discussed in Chapter 6.

Figure 1 shows the underlying dimensions of treatment ideologies (treatment roles and goals) arrayed in a typology, with the corresponding treatment ideology identified. (An earlier version of this typology was presented in Scheid 1994.) Some custodial providers act as agents of social control, and adhere to a coercive treatment ideology. They are likely to be found in inpatient settings, jails, or other institutions based on overt social control. Many of the providers interviewed had previously worked

Figure 1. Typology of Treament Ideologies

TREATMENT GOALS	ROLE OF THE PROVIDER		
	CUSTODIAL	SUPPORTIVE	FACILITATIVE
CONTROL	Coercive	Guardianship	Authorization
ADJUSTMENT	Supervisory	Caretaking	Reparenting
AUTONOMY	Enforcement	Normalization	Empowerment

on inpatient units, and described the coercive ideologies prevalent in "asylums."

> We put them in straps and leathers, we shot them up, and not just thorazine and haldol, but sodium phenithol . . . you're talking about a fifty-bed unit with six staff. It was like a jail. No treatment, no behavior problems, just march them in and march them out. (Female nurse case manager)

However, coercive treatment ideologies can also be found in outpatient settings (Estroff 1981; Goldin 1990; Teram 1991). Many of the providers in my research on outpatient commitment liked the law because it gave them more "control" over clients, it was a way to "twist their arm" and provided needed "leverage" in therapy (Scheid-Cook 1991; Scheid 1993). Providers who were critical of outpatient commitment felt that it didn't provide them with enough control over their clients; they "wished there were more teeth to enforce compliance." Case managers interviewed in the 1990s also sometimes took on more coercive ideologies, even though they saw their role as caring. "You have this caring relationship with them, and you just say, 'You have to do this'."

Alternatively, custodial providers may also work toward greater adjustment of the client, and hence adhere to a treatment ideology that is coercive rather than supervisory. These providers work to ensure that their clients do not get into trouble whether in the hospital, in the community, or at work, and view their clients as in need of a good deal of supervision. Many of the providers I interviewed about outpatient commitment felt that the law "worked" because it helped them to supervise their clients in the community more closely. More recently, some providers interviewed in the 1990s found they had to assume a supervisory role with their substance abuse clients, though generally they were not comfortable with this role.[3] A supervisory role was especially likely where the provider also functioned as a payee, or worked closely with the client's payee. A payee is the individual who controls the clients' financial resources, primarily because the clients have not acted responsibly with their money, or are likely to spend it on drugs or alcohol.

Custodial providers may also seek greater autonomy for their clients, within the confines of a given institutional space. These providers act as enforcers, giving the clients all possible freedom within a given set of organizational constraints and rules. For example, some providers work with clients who are so severely disabled either physically, emotionally, or cognitively, that they need ongoing custodial support, yet the clients are still able to exercise autonomous choice within that institutional space once their basic daily needs are met. In this case, providers act as agents of enforcement and ensure that clients do not stray too far afield. One case manager described the situation of being "an enforcer" in the following way:

> We are more willing to take chances with people . . . okay . . . you want to take your meds a little less often in front of us . . . okay . . . we'll give you a chance to do that, it's your life, not our life, but bear in mind, if you get sick and start acting weird, we are going to go to court against you, or call your probation officer. (Male MA case manager)

The client is granted autonomy, but the provider must enforce the boundaries around that sphere of autonomy.

Looking at the second column of the typology we have provider roles that entail a more supportive stance toward their clients. When dealing with clients who need control, these providers adhere to a treatment ideology described as guardianship. Such providers attempt to watch over their clients to help them eliminate the types of behavior that calls forth a coercive response such as forced medication, restraints, or commitment. Under a guardianship ideology, such responses would be used reluctantly, but would be viewed as necessary for the client. However, the provider tries to watch over the client and protect them from such harsh measures. Accordingly, the provider acts in a kind and benevolent manner. The following example comes from a provider's previous experience in an inpatient unit:

> I knew very soon I wasn't going to help anybody, I mean, we had someone who was on 2400 milligrams of thorazine a day . . . I wasn't going to change them, or help them. But I decided if I could be kind to them that's really something for them. Because the staff was abusive, and power hungry. To be in a supportive role is so much nicer. (Female nurse case manager)

Supportive providers are more comfortable seeking greater adjustment for their clients, and describe their treatment ideology as one of caretaking. Caretakers monitor medications and behavior, work to stabilize their clients in the community, and provide needed supports. Caretakers want to provide a haven for their clients either as an inpatient or outpatient, and will work within their organization to offer a variety of programs such as drop-in centers or clubhouses, that give clients a sense of belonging.

> This is the only place where some of them get physically touched—this is a place to get love—we're not going to put all these people back to work, back into the community. (Female rehab worker in a clubhouse)

A caretaking ideology seeks to develop settings where clients can be accepted for who they are. "We don't try to make them do things they don't want to, here they get what they need without a lot of stress." Caretakers see treatment as involving "a lot of support, encouragement, listening, and trust building." Their clients

> need the security of knowing somebody's there. I don't put a lot of energy into trying to change people. Often I don't say anything, just listening is needed. (Female MSW case manager)

Caretakers spend a lot of time ensuring that their clients' needs are met. Their goal is to "help them [the clients] become more functional in the community, deal with their hygiene, make sure they have food, that sort of thing, helping them to stay out of trouble with the law, find them places to live" (Female case manager).

Normalization refers to treatment techniques that result in behaviors characterized as socially normative (see Chapter 2). Under a normalization ideology the ultimate goal of treatment is community adjustment; clients are expected to resume normal lives in the community. Hence, much of the work of the provider oriented toward helping the client obtain income and housing that would enable them to live independently.

> I see how far people can go if they have a roof over their heads and their basic needs are cared for, then they can go and think about other things, like volunteer work. (Female rehab counselor)

Treatment often consists of socialization, or teaching clients social norms, needed skills, and ultimately the social control needed to fit into existing social roles. While supportive, the provider respects the client's autonomy.

> Just because you have a mental illness you don't lose the right to self-determination . . . We try to be as non-directive as possible in terms of making some life decisions . . . we would rather assist people in developing skills rather than force people to do what we want . . . we write plans for the client. (Male MSW supervisor and case manager)

Furthermore, providers adhering to a normalization ideology want their clients' "level of involvement with the mental health system to be less and less." In contrast, caretakers are more likely to see themselves playing a long-term role in their clients' lives; they "don't close charts anymore," since their clients are not expected to move on: "We're not going to put all these people back into the community."

The facilitative provider is most likely to see clients as partners in the treatment process. If the goal is control, the treatment ideology may be one of authorization. The provider works with the clients to teach them how the system works, to enlighten them as to the nature of their predicament and why others in society perceive them as needing social control. Facilitative providers are very likely to be uncomfortable with clients who need overt social control, but may find themselves in treatment settings where social control is an issue. Adolescent units and residential treatment settings often have clients who need to learn more social control, yet the role of the provider is more facilitative than supportive or coercive. Authorizers develop a trusting relationship with their clients, "so that they will do what they need." They may see medication as a means to control the symptoms of mental illness, but will work with their clients to educate them about their illness and need for medication.

If the goal of treatment is adjustment, facilitative providers often take on the role of quasiparents. Reparenting ideologies can be difficult to distinguish from caretaking ones, largely because of the wide variety of parenting styles. While "parents" do provide care, caretaking is viewed as a necessary evil and as only a temporary stage in the treatment process. They want the client to grow up and move out, and are critical of caretakers:

> Many people get into this field as caretakers. We do too much caretaking—
> we don't do enough to make them independent—teach them skills and ap-
> propriate behaviors, such as not picking your nose in public. (Female case
> manager)

Quasiparents argue that clients need fewer supportive services and more skills training; clients need to be taught to do things on their own. Rather than being walked through the system, clients need to be "pointed in the right direction" and if necessary given "a push." They need to learn certain behaviors that are necessary to functioning successfully or to adjust to the community.

> Reparenting is . . . we are going to teach you to clean your body, when you
> can do that you can go on a pass. Oops! You got drunk—you lose your priv-
> ileges for a month. I'm sorry, you still have to brush your teeth and clean your
> room. You learn a new skill, you can go out again . . . You learn ten new skills
> and you can move up a level. (Male MA case manager)

As this quote illustrates, quasiparents do not generally grant their clients as much autonomy as providers who advocate normalization or empowerment. The quasiparent knows what is best for the client, or what the client needs, and tries to get the client "to move in the *right* direction."

> I try to work with that person . . . working toward what they see as their goals . . . sometimes pushing them to feel what that is, influencing them in a direction that I think is best . . . and sometimes I think that's a little invasive, but I try to use my relationship with them to facilitate growth. (Male MSW case manager)

Reparenting does not engender the long-term dependency that the other treatment ideologies do; the client is expected to make progress and move on.

> I see us becoming more of a teaching model than a case-management model. We are not going to get people very far in life without teaching them skills. (Female MA case manager)

This quote is also illustrates the conflict between the ideals of care versus cure; providers want to see their clients' progress toward greater independence and less reliance on the mental health system. The ideologies of caretaking and reparenting reflect the conflict between the mandates to care for clients or to cure them. While both caretakers and parents adhere to the biopsychosocial model of mental health, they hold different views about their roles and the goals of treatment (reflecting the contradictions inherent in the model of community-based care) and were often critical of one another.

An empowerment treatment ideology seeks greater client control over mental health services, if not complete independence from the mental health system. Empowerment explicitly rejects the idea of clinical intervention (Paulson 1992). Instead it strives to enable clients to obtain those resources that give them control over their environments (Hasenfeld and Chesler 1989).

> I believe in being equal to clients. I mean they are the professionals in their lives, not me . . . and I think you need to empower clients, and if you (the client) are less of a person than I am, I'm not doing anybody any good. (Female MA case manager)

With the advent of empowerment ideologies, empowered clients are now called by the politically correct term "consumers."

> As a team we need to find ways to help the consumer participate in treatment, to take more responsibility and authority, with us as consultants rather than treatment that is *done* to them. (Male MSW case manager)

Rather than being socialized, or re-socialized, consumers are entrusted and authorized to assume control for their own lives and providers trust them to do so. Consumers set their own goals, and are encouraged to have a role in making decisions about service offerings and other critical organizational areas. As one provider described,

> I figure out what I can do for them, not to do it for them, but trying to get them to take responsibility for themselves. My background is really strong on consumer rights and responsibilities. I agree that people have a "right to fail" so you learn from your mistakes. We don't need to encourage dependence, but independence. I have been shocked at the lack of consumer involvement here in decision making. (Female MA case manager)

Ultimately, empowerment has the potential to challenge the status quo of mental health treatment and lead to radically new ways of understanding and approaching the treatment of mental illness. However, while much lip service has been paid to empowerment, most mental health organizations have not really involved consumers as autonomous agents in the organizational decision making processes. As one treatment team supervisor noted:

> I've seen a shift in talking about consumer involvement and client choice, and I'm not exactly sure how—but hopefully we can integrate that a little more by getting staff to value that more.

Providers who grant their clients autonomy are more likely to adhere to a normalization ideology. One provider who referred to himself as a "Shepherd" notes that

> it's my job to help persons think through what they want to accomplish, and how they might go about that, and so I see myself as herding now and then to help them maintain independent living. (Male MA case manager)

While such providers grant some autonomy, the client is not fully empowered or entitled to self-determination.

TREATMENT IDEOLOGIES IN PRACTICE

Having delineated the different treatment ideologies at the theoretical level, I will examine empirically the prevalence of these ideologies among providers and within specific organizational contexts, focusing on data obtained from in-depth interviews with providers in the two public sector mental health programs. Specific organizational practices and service interventions are "an enactment of the organization's practice ideology" (Hasenfeld 1992: 13). Different treatment ideologies will result in distinct treatment technologies and service interventions, and these have a direct impact on both client level outcomes and providers' evaluations of an organization's effectiveness. Diverse treatment ideologies point to considerable disagreement about organizational goals (referred to as goal incongruence) as well as to potential conflict between different groups of providers.

It is important to keep in mind that the treatment ideologies identified by the typology are ideal types (Weber 1946), that is, they are analytical constructs which help us to conceptualize empirical reality. Individuals will espouse elements of different ideologies, although it is possible to determine what kind of ideology a provider is most comfortable with, or has utilized in the past. In-depth interviews give a heightened sense of a provider's preferred, or actualized, treatment ideology. Often the critical incidents provide important clues as to how the provider prefers to act.

Table 3 presents the predominant treatment ideologies of the providers interviewed at the CARE (n=21) and SUPPORT (n=14). I eliminated one psychiatric technician from this analysis who worked on the crisis stabilization unit at CARE. Not surprisingly, this individual expressed a treatment ideology consistent with the need for social control even though she saw herself in a facilitative role. The majority of the providers are case managers, although some perform more psychosocial rehabilitation services such as housing or employment than case management per se. In addition to noting the organization in which the provider worked I also examine treatment ideology in terms of gender and professional role. All eight African-Americans worked with CARE and hence it would be difficult to protect their identity if race were also a factor.

Given that the research was collected in outpatient settings, very few providers adhered to primarily custodial roles, or sought control of their clients. Those that articulated some elements of these ideologies (n=3) were all male, over forty-five, and worked in a position where control, or a custodial role, was necessary (i.e., partial hospitalization—which is a day program—or a jail diversion program). Given that treatment ideologies are properties of a collectivity, these two mental health organizations exhibit cohesion around those treatment ideologies that are consistent with outpatient, community-based treatment, which is an important institutional demand. Community-based care postulates both adjustment and autonomy for clients' care as well as cure. Furthermore, providers can be both supportive and facilitative in their relations with clients. Often the role and the specific goal depend on the client.

> The endpoint is the best possible functioning and independence . . . symptom free, or at least have a level of symptoms that will let them get on with their life . . . there are times when we have to take control, but I think that is painful for staff, so we avoid taking too much control and try to give it back when that's possible. (Male MSW supervisor)

Table 3. Analysis of Treatment Ideologies (percentages; n=35 providers)

TREATMENT IDEOLOGY	ORGANIZATION		GENDER		OCCUPATION			
	Care (14)	Support (21)	Male (14)	Female (21)	Case-Mgr (22)	Nurse (7)	Rehab (4)	Other (2)
Custodial								
Coercive (0)								
Supervisory (0)								
Enforcement (0)								
Supportive								
Guardianship (0)								
Care-taking (9)	14%	33%	7%	38%	14%	71%	—	50%
Normalization (14)	36	38	43	33	27	29	100	50
Facilitative								
Authorization (1)	0	5.0	7.0		5.0			
Reparenting (7)	29	14	29	14	32			
Empowerment (5)	21	10	14	14	23			

Generally, the first treatment goal for a client is adjustment. Most providers hope that clients will move to greater autonomy and self-determination, although some never talk about clients gaining control over their lives. While the ideologies can be thought of as a continuum (with greater freedom at the ends of the axis) providers do not view all ideologies as equally valid. Thus there is potential for interorganizational conflict.

In both mental health organizations, more providers adhered to a normalization treatment ideology (36 percent at SUPPORT and 38 percent at CARE); followed by 29 percent of those at SUPPORT being more likely to articulate a reparenting ideology and 33.3 percent of those at CARE holding a caretaking ideology. This difference may be due to gender as opposed to organizational philosophy. Twenty-eight percent of the providers interviewed at CARE were male, and 57 percent of the providers at SUPPORT were male (which matches the overall demographic distribution at these sites); overall 60 percent of the providers were female and 40 percent were male. Male providers were more likely to espouse a normalization ideology (43 percent), followed by reparenting (29 percent). Female providers were most likely to adhere to a caretaking ideology (38 percent) followed by normalization (33 percent).

In terms of professional backgrounds, all of the providers who saw their roles as facilitators were case managers, which is not surprising, given their role duties. Providers who adhered to normalization were more likely to be case managers (27 percent), or rehabilitation workers (28 percent). In large part due to their professional training and holistic orientation, nurses were more likely to adhere to a caretaking model (71 percent); the one male caretaker was also a nurse—the only male nurse in the sample. This supports much of the literature on the caregiving orientation of the nursing profession (Chambliss 1996).

Although the data are merely exploratory, they demonstrate the ways in which providers have "enacted" the broader institutional demands for community-based care. The majority of the providers adhere to treatment ideologies that are consistent with the principles of community-based care: caretaking, reparenting, normalization, and empowerment. There is evidence of conflict between institutional demands for care as opposed to cure, normalization as opposed to empowerment. Case managers were far more likely to assume a facilitative role, nurses a supportive role. We might therefore expect case managers and therapists to be more frustrated by the caretaking needs of their clients, and some evidence of this was evident in the quote cited above.

We can also expect treatment ideologies to change over time within specific organizational settings in response to the changing institutional demands for care described in the previous chapter. The surveys at CARE I conducted in 1998 and 2000 used two open-ended questions to determine the treatment ideology of providers. First, I asked providers to identify their treatment objectives or goals: "In your opinion, given your existing caseload, what constitutes successful care or treatment of a client?" Second, I asked them to describe their role with clients: "I must assume the role of a _____ (please provide a descriptor for how you see your role in the relationship with your clients)." From the responses to these two questions I categorized provider's treatment ideologies. Unfortunately, not all providers answered both questions, and many providers described their role in terms of their occupational role (i.e., nurse or social worker) so the data are limited. Although the providers' brief responses to these two questions do not reflect the complexity of their treatment ideologies, this analysis does give us some insight into changes in treatment ideologies over time.

I first look at changes from 1998 to 2000 in providers' descriptions of successful care or treatment because they were more developed than their descriptions of their role. The responses were easily classified into the three categories described earlier: control, adjustment, and autonomy. In 1998, twenty-six providers completed well-developed answers describing their role, and in 2000, twenty-seven providers did. Control goals emphasized stability: providers wanted their clients "stabilized on medications, educated about illness and medications" (1998: #62). Several providers mentioned "management in a facility." Other providers talked more directly about "client compliance" as a treatment goal (2000: #54). Adjustment meant:

> Linking clients with all possible services, the ability to ensure follow through and satisfaction with services, the client is able to live in a place on their own and have their basic needs met. (1998: #30)

Autonomy was achieved if the client moved to greater independence:

> If they demonstrate less dependence on the system and move to a more independent living environment, or become an active participant in their treatment. (2000: #69)

The number of providers indicating their treatment goal was client adjustment remained stable at 17 in 1998, and 16 in 2000. However, the number of providers indicating coercive treatment goals dropped from seven to two, while the number of providers seeking greater autonomy for their clients increased from two to nine.

Table 4 compares changes in the treatment objectives of providers at CARE between 1990 and 2000. In 1990, normalization was the most prevalent treatment ideology at CARE (36 percent), in 2000 caretaking (28 percent) and reparenting (28 percent) are slightly more prevalent than normalization (24 percent). Providers were somewhat less likely to articulate empowerment in 2000, although they did seek greater autonomy for

Table 4. Changes in Treatment Objectives at CARE (%)

	1990 (N=14)	2000 (N=25)
TREATMENT IDEOLOGY		
Caretaking	14%	28%
Normalization	36	24
Authorization	0	4
Reparenting	29	28
Empowerment	21	16

their clients. This may be a reflection of an increasingly bureaucratic system of care that has disempowered providers.

CONCLUDING POINTS

I begin with the caveat that the typology of treatment ideologies developed in this chapter is not fixed and is not intended to represent all potential ideologies about the treatment of those with serious mental illness. It is historically framed by the institutional expectations and demands (rational myths) about the treatment and care of individuals with serious mental illness that prevailed in the 1980s and 1990s, (when the data were collected). As with ideal types in general (Weber 1946), when the institutional environment changes, the range of potential ideologies may change as well to reflect new conditions and demands. (See Scott et. al. 2000 for an excellent discussion of the effects of changing institutional environments on health care.)

Given that the institutional environment dictates psychosocial rehabilitation, and case management is viewed as the best means to achieve community integration for clients with severe mental illness, it is not surprising that the two mental health organizations studied exhibited treatment ideologies largely consistent with these institutional demands. Yet within the spacious framework of psychosocial rehabilitation, providers did enact more specific ideologies with differing emphasis on the degree of autonomy granted to the clients, and the type of assistance the provider offered to help clients meet these goals. Furthermore, treatment ideologies were clearly properties of the treatment team, or organizational unit in which providers worked. They were generally described in terms of the way "we do things" around here, and "different agencies do have different perspectives on what their obligations are to clients." Thus, providers articulated instances when their own preferences conflicted with those of the wider group or organization.

There was not much evidence of homogenization. At neither site did providers receive much informal indoctrination; instead most "imported" their models of care. This was particularly evident at SUPPORT, where the majority of providers had MSWs from a nearby university. However, there is as much variability in specific treatment ideologies at SUPPORT as there is at CARE, where many providers lacked a master's degree and came from different educational and occupational backgrounds. This similarity in the type and variability of treatment ideology underscores the importance of the institutional environment, the two organizations' commitment to providing innovative, community-based care, and the degree of autonomy granted to mental health workers in these two sites.

While the treatment ideologies espoused at SUPPORT and CARE are consistent with broad institutional mandates for community-based care, the potential for conflict over the best means to achieve such care remains. In particular, providers who advocate empowerment and greater consumer control are in conflict with those providers who see clients as needing greater direction and guidance (or even control). Evidence showed the dilemma faced by providers who must choose between merely managing the care provided to a client and moving clients along in their development. Few of the providers felt their clients needed therapy; instead they viewed their clients' needs from within the framework of community-based care. Case management was viewed as the primary means to provide necessary care, and was not seen as merely a means to manage care. Individuals with serious mental illnesses need a broad array of community supports, and providers recognized the critical role they played coordinating those services. Many had also been socialized to believe (or had learned from experience) that therapy by itself simply did not work with clients with severe mental illnesses. One MSW provider stated quite bluntly that her previous counseling sessions with schizophrenics "were one hour of torture." However, some providers felt that they relied on medication too heavily and that more therapy was needed.

There was some diversity of treatment ideologies within each organization, indicating the potential for conflict over service offerings and treatment technologies. At both organizations providers disagreed over the need for supported employment versus day treatment programs, extended community outreach versus specialized programs for particular client groups, medication compliance versus the right to refuse medications, and the feasibility of consumer-run services. These choices are necessitated by restricted resources. With managed care, the restriction of services forces providers to make hard choices about different service offerings. (In the words of one provider, "Taxpayers aren't willing to support more programs such as this.") Furthermore, those services which demonstrate proven outcomes are given the greatest preference. The outcome of debates over the type of community mental health care that works best will be determined in part by the salience and support for the different treatment ideologies described in this chapter, as well as the new ones that may arise.

NOTES

1. In their study of two psychiatric hospitals, Strauss et al. (1964) identified three philosophies: somatotherapeutic (or organic), psychotherapeutic, and milieu or sociotherapeutic (environmental). It is clear these philosophies correspond to the biomedical, psychosocial, and social models described in the previous chapter. Strauss et al. (1964) also described a polarity between ideologies that emphasized treatment, as opposed to custodial care, arguing that the problems of chronic illness required moral (as opposed to merely medical) considerations. In a later work Strauss et al. (1985) focus on how chronic illness changes the practice of medicine and care. Kleinman (1988) has also argued that the medical model is inappropriate for chronic illness.

2. McDonald (1991) also argues that in order for treatment to be effective there must be a match between a client and his/her provider in terms of their domain assumptions. As noted by Broman et al. (1994) a mismatch between the goals and expectations of the provider and the client may well lead to poor outcomes.

3. It is interesting that both CARE and SUPPORT used outpatient commitment for clients with substance abuse problems.

4 Rationed Mental Health Care

Changing Provider Roles

I am discouraged because I feel as if there are business forces, or political forces, beyond my reach that are dictating the way I am going to run my professional life, and I feel it's only going to get worse. (PhD psychiatrist in private practice)

Health care has undergone profound institutional change (Alexander and D'Aunno 1990; Light 1997; Scott et al. 2000) as delivery systems, including mental health, have been transformed by managed care. In 1989, the Institute of Medicine defined managed care as

a set of techniques used by or on behalf of purchasers of health care benefits to manage health care costs by influencing patient care decision making through case-by-case assessment of the appropriateness of care prior to its provision. (Wells et. al., 1995: 57).

Managed care is a revolutionary change from a provider-driven to a buyer-driven system of health care (Light 1997). Beigel et al. (1997: 309) liken the institutional force of managed care to "a supersonic plane announced by a sonic boom." While there has been a great deal of uncertainty about the impact of managed care on the delivery of mental health services and client level outcomes, "it is clear that mental health care has become a commodity under managed care, and that cost is the principle mechanism for assigning quality at present" (Manderscheid et al. 1999: 412).

Managed care represents a response to the wider normative demand for technical rationality and efficiency. Meyer (1990) conceptualizes this process of rationalization in terms of the commodity model of organizations (in opposition to the traditional bureaucratic model). The bureaucratic model postulates that organizational structures shape efficiency outcomes. The commodity model reverses this process: organizational structures are *outcomes* of efficiency constraints. Furthermore, rationality is not so much a matter of finding the appropriate means to a given end (the

63

bureaucratic model), but of achieving given ends, such as the accumulation of wealth, profit, or saving public investment (the commodity model). Consequently, efficiency and rationality "are synonymous, or nearly so . . . organizational structure is the outcome of rationality/efficiency imperatives, not the other way around" (Meyer 1990: 209). Heydeband (1990) refers to the technical-rational approaches to organizational decision-making as the new managerialism, characterized by its blending of productive and administrative functions. Consistent with Heydeband's (1990) analysis of academia, the new managerialism in health care emerged in response to the perceived crisis of rising health care costs, relying upon computer assisted analysis and is results-oriented.

The pivotal forces propelling the movement to managed care in the 1980s were financial, namely, reduced government support for public sector health care and escalating costs in the private sector (Bazelon Center 1995; Mechanic 1999). Although managed care affords an opportunity to reorganize mental health care systems and improve the delivery of care (Boyle and Callahan 1995), its key institutional logic is cost-containment.

> Managed care emerged as an effort to introduce cost as a crucial element in clinical decision making and health care policy. Managed care involves accounting for every dollar spent. (Schreter et al. 1994: xiii)

The primary means to control costs is to limit services; consequently, many are concerned that managed care will restrict access to care and will result in lower levels or poorer qualities of care (Schlesinger 1995). The contradiction posed by managed care is most concisely articulated by the often-heard refrain that managed care is not about managing care, but about managing costs.

The change to managed care results in a paradigm shift when a rational business ethic and corresponding system of bureaucratic control are imposed on organizations that had previously operated on the basis of a professionally determined moral foundation and ambiguous goals (Schelesinger and Gray 1999; Soderfeldt et al. 1996). Organizations and providers must meet the primary goal of cost-containment (whether for profit-based systems or to save "scarce" public funds), by determining the most effective means to achieve these financially determined goals, and then monitoring performance to ensure that services are delivered in a cost-efficient manner. In short, the current requirements for efficiency, measurable outcomes, and cost-containment constitute an institutional demand to which mental health care organizations must conform if they are to attain and maintain legitimacy in an environment in which mental health care has become a commodity. Many writers focus on outcome assessment as a principal characteristic of managed care (Martin and Kettner 1997), and, while performance accountability may well be a good thing, it must be remembered that the measurement of performance is determined by the fundamental goal of cost-containment. In terms of mental health care services, the delivery systems or treatment practices are expected to produce those treatment outcomes that result in a financial return. This is a difficult institutional demand to implement when clients' health care problems are chronic, providers disagree about appropriate treatment (Schlesinger and Gray 1999), and the primary costs of inadequate mental health are born by the wider community (Mechanic 1999).

The institutional demand for technical rationality is not limited to health care; all institutional spheres (manufacturing, education, government, social services) respond to the demand that organizations become "lean" machines that produce goods and/or services that meet the goal of profit or cost-containment. However, the institutional logic of "lean" production conflicts with professionally based logics of mental health care. The conflict is overt. "By design, managed care is intended to alter clinical practices" (Schlesinger and Gray 1999: 441). As in other institutional spheres, deprofessionalization is one of the outcomes of the new managerialism (Heydeband 1990). Mental health practitioners experience this conflict in terms of "ethical dilemmas" as they struggle to defend established treatment practices in the face of institutional demands for cost-containment and performance-based outcomes (Fletcher 1998; Galambos 1999; Scheid 2002; Ware et al. 2000).

This chapter examines the effect the commodification of mental health care on the work of mental health care providers. The core argument is that the ideology of managed care, which embraces cost-containment as its ultimate goal, is inherently incompatible with that of community-based care, which is generated by professionals. Community-based care relies on a social rather than a medical model of illness and treatment, and it embraces a biopsychosocial philosophy of care.[1] Although serious mental illness is viewed as a disease requiring medication in many cases, psychosocial rehabilitation is the primary treatment modality of community-based care. Psychosocial rehabilitation emphasizes community integration rather than merely the relief of symptoms (which is the medically defined treatment goal). The goal of psychosocial rehabilitation is to develop the adaptive capacities of the client in the community, foster the community's attitudes of tolerance and respect (i.e., combat stigma) and provide the continuum of care needed by clients with severe, chronic mental illness (Bockoven 1972). For those with acute illnesses, community-based care emphasizes prevention and the achievement of optimum mental heath and functioning. Managed care, with its emphasis on cost-containment and short-term therapeutic goals, adheres to a treatment modality more in keeping with a medical model of illness: when one is "sick," one receives some sort of medication or short-term treatment until one is "recovered." Treatment goals are set in terms of short-term improvements in functional ability. Furthermore, medical care is provided by organizations with a business focus, and governed by a technocratic rationality.

Currently, providers are seeking to integrate managed care principles into delivery systems organized around the tenets of community-based care, and mental health professionals are struggling to define managed care in such a way that community care principles are safeguarded (Carpinello et al. 1998; Ogles et al. 1998). However, providers must negotiate between contradictory institutional demands in their work practices. These contradictions are experienced as a series of ethical dilemmas. In addition, managed care inevitably results in a higher level of external (i.e., third party) control over clinical work practices. Consequently, providers are likely to feel that they are not performing their jobs appropriately. Their experience of frustration, inauthenticity, and emotional dissonance is likely to result in higher levels of job dissatisfaction and burnout.

First, I describe managed care and how it works, and then I consider the impact of managed care on mental health services, in terms of the ways in which managed care has changed the role of the provider and the resulting ethical dilemmas providers face in attempting to manage care within the confines of a commodity model. I rely upon accounts of managed care provided in the literature, my interviews with providers in private practice, and my case study of a small, private nonprofit outpatient agency, Venture, that moved very early (in 1989) to managed care. Venture provides training to approximately twenty psychiatric residents at a nearby university, and is staffed by eight psychiatrists, one nurse, three master's level therapists, two clinical case managers, and the clinical care director with a MSW, who also maintains her own caseload. Providers at Venture have worked together in close proximity for a long time with little turnover and view themselves as a family. I conducted a series of in-depth and focus group interviews at Venture in 1998. Earlier, in 1996, Venture had contracted with the county to provide mental health care to over two thousand Medicaid clients, and thus exemplified one of the ways in which managed care has eliminated the distinction between private and public systems of mental health care.

HOW MANAGED CARE WORKS

Managed care began to have an impact on mental health services in the 1980s. It emerged first in the private sector and is currently being implemented by most public mental health care systems (Mechanic 1999). As described by Tuttle and Woods (1997: 1), managed mental health care has evolved as a system of cost-containment, research-based treatment plans, and setting standards for services and payment. Mental health care had frequently been "carved-out" of basic health care plans and was initially left unmanaged, or else managed by specialty mental health care clinics. There has been tremendous growth in for-profit "behavioral health care" organizations. (The term "behavioral" refers to the combination of substance and mental health care, and is often used in place of the term "mental health.") Kihlstrom (1997) studied 106 managed "behavioral" care organizations from 1990 to 1994 and found a turbulent field with an increasing number of mergers and consolidations; the majority of the firms were for-profit and were owned by insurance companies or managed care corporations.

There are a number of mechanisms by which mental health care is managed (Mechanic 1999), including gatekeeping (where access to specialty mental health care is controlled by requirements for referral from a primary care provider); precertification or utilization review (where services must be authorized before a client can receive them); concurrent review or case management (ongoing review of treatment at regular intervals, and capitation (where a predetermined fee is paid for a defined benefit with a given amount of time). Capitation provides the greatest incentive for improved cost-control and efficiency, although it is very difficult to arrive at an accurate prospective payment scheme for mental illness, especially those conditions that are chronic and/or severe (Minkoff and Pollack 1997). Venture utilizes case rates for capitation. In 1998 these were set at $1,000 per client per year, but the rates do not include the costs of medication, which Venture is able to provide because of the connections the university-affiliated psychiatrists have with pharmaceutical companies.

Private mental health care is principally funded by employer-based insurance plans. Driven by both the complementary desires of employers to keep costs down, and of insurers to keep profits high, private sector health care quickly became managed. By 1995, nearly three-fourths of U.S. workers received managed health care, either through a health maintenance organization (HMO), a preferred provider organization (PPO), or point of service plan (Jensen et al. 1997). Most private plans provide some coverage for mental health and/or substance abuse services, but the coverage is generally more limited than coverage for physical health care (Buck and Umland 1997; Jensen et al. 1998). In a recent survey of employer-sponsored health plans Buck et al. (1999) found a slight increase in the proportion of health plans that covered mental health or substance abuse services and a slight decrease in the use of limits on mental health benefits.

In contrast to the private sector, public sector mental health care benefits have always been "managed" to some extent (Lazarus and Pollock 1997). That is, providers were expected to meet the needs of geographically defined populations with limited resources. Consequently, cost-containment already was a critical component in the institutional environment of public sector mental health care. Public mental health care is financed primarily through Medicaid (need-based health care for the poor and disabled) and Medicare (universal coverage for the elderly). The needs of in-dividuals with chronic or long-term mental health needs are generally supported by Medicaid funds. Medicaid provides for basic hospital and outpatient services, and states are able to develop more comprehensive services with federal subsidies (Mechanic 1999). Consequently, benefits and the availability of services vary from state to state.

Medicaid funding exemplifies the contradiction between unlimited de-mand for health care and limited resources; only by limiting access to care can delivery systems ensure health care is available to everyone (Freund and Hurley 1995: 476). While provisions for enrollment in managed care plans for Medicaid recipients have been available for some time, enroll-ment in such plans was limited until the early 1990s, when managed care "exploded" in the private sector (Freund and Hurley 1995). Many states subsequently turned to managed care as a means to control costs and pro-vide for better system coordination (Mechanic 1999; Schlesinger and Gray 1999). There is remarkable (and perhaps distressing) variation in state plans to manage behavioral health (Hanson and Huskamp 2001; Mander-scheid and Henderson 2000). Some have attained at best modest success while others have failed (Croze 2001). Utilization and concurrent review have been the most common forms of public sector managed mental health care, though systems are increasingly turning to capitation to control costs.

Managed care controls costs primarily by limiting clients' access to ser-vices and by limiting their utilization of more costly services by encourag-ing them to use less costly services. In order to determine the cost effectiveness of a given treatment, managed care systems must assess em-pirically verifiable "success," or outcomes. Mental health treatment must be "medically necessary"; increasingly, managed care companies will only reimburse services that have been scientifically validated as efficacious. One managed care consultant (Schreter et al. 1994: 57) describes utilization review as *ideally* allowing for:

1. Independent and scientific determination of the efficacy of a procedure.
2. Independent and scientific determination of the appropriateness of in-dicators for such a procedure.
3. Independently determined indicators that have been reduced to no more than a fifteen-minute question-and-answer telephone review or written questionnaire.

An important obstacle to evaluating managed mental health care is the dif-ficulty in evaluating treatment effectiveness. The managed care consultant quoted above stated, "To remove the emperor's clothes, *no* utilization re-view program has workable criteria for reviewing outpatient care" (ibid.: 58). As shown in previous chapters, there is little consensus among providers about the etiology of mental illness or its appropriate treatments. Not only is it difficult to define the nature of the problem, but different types of treatment work with different types of clients. In terms of chronic and severe mental illness, clients may not show noticeable signs of improvement, even within excellent programs (Mechanic and Schlesinger, 1993; Mechanic et al. 1995), making it far more difficult to determine standards for medical necessity (Manderscheid and Henderson 2000). Moreover, client confidentiality limits collection of, and access to, data. Yet managed care companies must rely on the assessment of client outcomes, and propel the development of a scientifically (as opposed to professionally based) system of treatment and practice guidelines.[2] A critical component of any managed care entity is an adequate information system that can organize client-level and provider-level data to allow for some assessment of treatment outcomes.

Managed care has resulted in fewer inpatient care episodes and reduced hospital stays and has thus reduced the overall costs of mental health care, since inpatient care is more costly than outpatient care (Durham 1998; Manderscheid and Henderson 2000). The price paid for these savings is restricted access (Weisman et al. 2000). Furthermore, most managed care plans do not cover chronic mental illness in their standard benefits packages, and the amount of money generally allocated for mental health services in not considered sufficient for adequate treatment (Iglehart 1996; Manderscheid and Henderson 2000). In addition, providers often face pressure from their managed care organization to provide even less treatment than what is covered by a patient's benefits plan, especially when fees are capitated. Mechanic and McAlpine (1999) argue that managed care has produced a "democratization" of care where everyone gets a similar level of services and those with greater needs (chronic mental illness) do not get the services they need. With reduced inpatient stays, individuals with chronic care needs have higher rates of readmissions. While the Health Maintenance Act of 1973 required plans to provide up to twenty outpatient sessions per year, the criteria of medical necessity and measurable outcomes within a reasonable time frame has resulted in a reliance upon short-term therapy, group sessions, and psychiatric medications.

The data I collected from private practice providers illustrate how practices have changed with managed care. Providers reported that anywhere from 50 to 80 percent of their clients were covered by some form of managed care and that they dealt with on average four to five different managed care companies. One-third of the providers felt that managed care had influenced the types of clients they served, and 40 percent felt it had changed the types of services they provide as well. One MSW stated, "It has changed the type of therapy I do. It's more here and now and outcome oriented." All had experienced pressures to provide short-term therapy, as illustrated by quotes from three different doctoral psychologists.

They say there is no difference in how you treat these people. It's all short-term.

They try to convince me that long-term treatment doesn't do anything better than short-term treatment.

Managed care forces therapists to only be able to do short-term stress reduction, and has inhibited more ongoing work on personality patterns and long-term change.

It is interesting that managed care companies try to influence the treatment practices of even PhD psychologists. Along with the emphasis on short-term therapy, managed care companies also stress the use of medications as medications have a known efficacy and are relatively cheaper than therapy. Luhrmann (2000) describes how managed care has undermined psychotherapy and legitimated psychopharmacology. Yet, as one psychiatrist argued, this change in treatment orientation is not fully warranted by the existing state of scientific knowledge.

It has driven us away from therapy to doing meds . . . The way it has changed practice in general, I think, is the tension between assuming a diagnosis means criteria for medical necessity. There are 200 schools of therapeutic thought; there are 15 different psychotropic meds, and many antidepressives. And the data is not in to say which is right. It's just an acute care benefit, to handle a crisis and that's it.

Many providers find themselves in the position of having to "sell clinical services" and decisions about care are increasingly made by business and financial specialists rather than clinical directors (Tuttle and Wood 1997). In private practice providers have experienced sometimes dramatic reductions in their reimbursements for services; one MA counselor stated, "It's demoralizing and demeaning to get $35 for sessions." Rates are set at a fraction of the fee-for-service equivalent. Freund and Hurley (1995: 482) report that this fraction is typically 95 percent for Medicaid enrollees. Private clinicians report fractions that are much lower. Tuttle and Wood (1997) and Moffic (1997) found that reimbursement levels were 30 percent below those of traditional fee-for-service. One female MSW said:

I get less money, much less money to be on panels, and then, also, the amount of paperwork, oh Lordy, it's starting to look like the county bureaucracy.

Another MSW felt she "works harder for less money. I spend a lot more time on the phone, maybe an hour a day." Other providers reported working longer hours; one psychotherapist increased his weekly work-hour over fifteen years from the average forty hours per week to sixty–seventy hours in order to maintain his income. The providers in my sample reported that managed care paid at least 20 percent less than traditional fee for service. Not all of the providers felt that the reduced fees were bad, one MSW said:

> the only good thing that managed care has done is it has made people more accountable for what they do. There was a tremendous amount of waste and abuses . . . lowering the fees for doctors and therapists is not a bad thing.

Several providers and provider groups removed themselves from managed care contracts and advertised that they no longer worked with managed care companies. Some providers said there would "always be patients who can pay out of pocket." Others found they could offer lower fees and still come out ahead, since they saved on administrative overhead and on time lost arguing with managed care companies. However, opting out of managed care meant denying care to those who cannot afford to pay for services. Ware et al. (2000) found concern among mental health care providers that managed care would exacerbate existing inequalities as well as racist assumptions about who can benefit from therapy.

In fact, one of the benefits of managed care described by providers in private practice was that it had widened access to some degree. As Mechanic and McAlpine (1999) also note, with managed care more people are able to get mental health services (and parity plays some role here). Providers noted that managed care had "allowed less financially solvent patients to come into private therapy" and that they were seeing more "blue collar clients." However, these clients often had more severe problems and providers were frustrated with the limits managed care placed on their client's treatment.

Increasingly, managed care entities are utilizing case rates, where a flat rate is paid for each client for one year of care. These rates vary but the average rate of $200 to $500 per year is widely considered to be very low (Moffic 1997; Tuttle and Woods 1997). In order to control costs, public care entities and area authorities contract out many of their services to private clinics agencies and clinics, or else privatize some of their own services. Yet it remains to be seen if managed care can indeed integrate systems of care that have historically been fragmented, or guarantee provision of the types of coordinated health and social services needed by clients with chronic conditions requiring long-term care. As one psychiatrist articulated:

> The buzzwords of managed care [are] "seamless, integrated systems of care" and I'm part of that. But there is a long way to go before it's seamless . . . it's more fragmented now, and I think that's from managing the dollars and not the care.

In terms of care for those with severe mental illnesses, there has been widespread concern that "an already vulnerable population" will be placed at "even greater risk for being managed toward the bottom line rather than toward improved client outcomes" (Durham 1995: 117). A focus on cost-containment of necessity results in the reduction of services deemed less costly, intensive, and long term; as one clinician reports, "crucial longer-term follow-up is often denied by cost reviewers" (Schreter et al. 1994: 62). Yet those with serious mental illness require long-term and integrated services (Mechanic 1994, 1999), and are generally disadvantaged under managed care systems (Bazelon Center 1995; Mechanic and McAlpine 1999; Morrissey 1999). Of critical importance is the motive behind a given managed care entity: is it to manage care (seeking to improve outcomes as well as care) or to manage reimbursements so as to reduce costs? Profit-driven organizations are motivated by the management of costs, while nonprofit organizations may still view their mission in terms of the management of care.

THE REALITY OF MANAGED MENTAL HEALTH CARE

Many mental health professionals believe that managed care has the potential to provide for the types of integrated service systems envisioned by proponents of community-based care. According to the Institute of Medicine (1997: 47):

> The introduction of managed care into already existing public-sector service systems represents a reorganization of service delivery and creates opportunities to address many limitations of the current systems of care.

Unmanaged systems have historically been characterized as leading to a lack of patient access, a lack of accountability, and a lack of coordination and continuity (Hoge et al. 1994). Case management, Assertive Community Treatment and local mental health authorities are all strategies which were employed to overcome the problems of fragmented and uncoordinated delivery systems (Dill and Rochefort 1989). Managed care is seen by some to have resulted from the failures of these earlier attempts to coordinate care (Boyle and Callahan 1995).

While fee-for-service reimbursement makes it difficult for the provider to coordinate care, capitation can potentially allow payment to be made for what each client needs. Hawthorne and Hough (1997: 217) acknowledge that "capitation-based systems lend themselves to abuse by failure to provided needed and necessary services and resources." Capitation is also a problematic approach for clients with long-term care needs and serious mental illnesses because of "the difficulty of predicting with any accuracy their future utilization patterns" (Mechanic 1999: 158). Manderscheid and Henderson (2000) state that few states have set capitation rates correctly, in part because these rates have been based on past expenditures and mental health systems have historically been underfunded.

Venture is a good example of how capitated managed care can work to the advantage of public sector clients. As noted earlier, Venture provides care to Medicaid clients by virtue of a contract with the county; the majority of these clients are indigent and have serious mental illnesses. The case rate is generous, at $1,000 plus the cost of medication. The managed care contract with the county stipulates that clients are to receive no more than ten hours of therapy or ten outpatient visits. Venture also provides care to private-pay clients (about 60 percent of the client census) whose care is reimbursed by a variety of different insurance plans and is largely managed. It is interesting to note that public sector clients had an advantage over many of the private-pay clients because private sector managed care rarely authorized ten visits. As one therapist articulated in the focus group interview:

> Those without insurance get a better shake, at least in this clinic, than those with insurance. They (the uninsured) get at least ten visits; those with insurance rarely get that.

In addition to improvements in the coordination of care, the emphasis upon the assessment of outcomes can lead to clearer standards for treatment and a more effective matching of services to individual client needs (Mechanic et al. 1995). Several providers in private practice felt that managed care had produced a needed accountability; one psychologist felt that managed care had made "therapists think more about outcomes, progress, and patient satisfaction." A PhD psychoanalyst felt it was good she now had to produce "measurable results;" another MA therapist felt managed care had "produced more goal setting and follow through."

There is also potential that managed care will produce more flexible, innovative treatment approaches. As one MSW at Venture remarked, "It [managed care] encourages you to use the most effective model of therapy," and another MSW therapist felt that managed care had the potential "to heighten a clinician's creativity and responsibility." The Medicaid freedom-of-choice (1915b) waivers do allow for the development of alternative approaches to treatment (Bazelon Center 1995), though I am not aware of any research that has described or assessed such innovations.

Managed care places more emphasis on group therapy and the use of interdisciplinary treatment teams or group practices to provide care (Alperin and Phillips 1997). Providers have found that the formation of multidisciplinary treatment practices allows them to survive in the managed care environment. The majority of referrals go to preferred-provider groups (Tuttle and Woods 1997) whose economies of scale are favored by managed care firms. Providers find that grouping allow them to economize on the administrative overhead associated with managed care. Psychiatrists and psychologists must join such multidisciplinary practices if they are to maintain any kind of independent practice. Providers in private practices are dependent on referrals from managed care entities who review the number of denials for treatment, readmissions, client outcomes, therapy approach, and costs of care in deciding which providers to keep on their panels (i.e., lists of providers from whom a client can obtain authorized services). One MSW stated, "We are moving toward more group practices; the individual therapist who hangs out a shingle are going to be few and far between." In large speciality managed care firms (with 20,000 to 35,000 providers) nearly 80 percent of referrals are going to only 20 percent of the providers (Tuttle and Woods 1997)—mostly those in multidisciplinary group practices.

Because of the limitations on outpatient visits with managed care, Venture has turned to group treatment approaches. At the time of my interviews, Venture ran eight different groups for over one hundred fifty clients. These groups were not viewed as effective as individual psychotherapy, and providers remarked that clients were not motivated to attend the groups. Consequently, providers lost time tracking down clients who failed to show up. At the same time Venture still maintained a policy that allowed for both walk-in and emergency appointments and provided assistance with transportation (bus tokens) for clients in need.

The potential for managed care to improve mental health services exists only within the limited framework governed by standards of cost-containment and efficiency. With managed care, mental health has become a commodity and mental health care organizations are in the business of providing a low-cost service to their customers, whether they have private insurance or are supported by public funds. According to one clinician:

outpatient psychological services have traditionally been organized around the biopsychosocial model . . . clinicians are under pressure to abandon it (the biopyschosocial model) in favor of treatment based on efficacy. Efficacy can be translated as clinical care that takes into account cost-effectiveness and the bottom line. (Schreter et al. 1994: 64)

Another private clinician fears that "we will sacrifice the psychosocial aspect of the biopsychosocial model" (Schreter et al. 1994: 115). Both public and private organizations measure client care in terms of short-term changes in functional ability, and utilize those treatments with known clinical efficacy—primarily psychiatric medications. Furthermore, there is greater reliance upon psychiatric medication as opposed to more intensive forms of therapy or skills training (Alperin and Phillips 1997; Mechanic 1999) . Consequently, the goals of treatment have changed to reflect a medical rather than a social, model of mental illness.

Neugeboren (1999) provides a poignant analysis of the mental health system and opportunities for meaningful recovery. He has also written about his brother, Robert, who has a serious mental illness and has spent his entire life in various mental institutions (Neugeboren 1997). Neugeboren (1999) investigates the range of community alternatives available, and describes the experiences of a number of consumers who have indeed "recovered" and are now providing other consumers with innovative programs. Recovery (as measured by improvements in functional ability and decreased symptomatology) is certainly possible, and medications do in fact help many individuals. But recovery requires a range of community supports and environments that are open and accommodating to those with multiple needs.

> If, like my brother, individuals with long-term histories of madness and of institutionalization—along with homelessness, poverty, drug abuse, prostitution, incarcerations, and violent acts perpetrated and/or endured— suddenly, through the agency of medication, come back literally to their senses, what do they do then? If medications suddenly and miraculously alleviate symptoms—even their causes—what do these individuals do in the next hour, day, month, or year of their lives? What do they do, for starters, with regard to the basics of life—food, clothing, shelter, education, finances, and employment? What do they do with their desires for friendship and love? What do they do with their fears and sorrows? (Neugeboren 1999: 304)

Mental health care providers have been meeting their clients' various needs, ranging from housing to emotional support. Managed care limits caregiving to medication, and does not worry about the ongoing social support needs of clients who are able to recover.

With its emphasis on cost-containment, managed care must limit services to clients (Iglehart 1996) and offer less intensive services. The greatest impact of these limitations will be felt by those clients with long-term care needs and chronic mental illnesses for whom "cost sharing is likely to impose barriers to care" (Mechanic and Schlesinger 1993: 125). While some argue that short-term therapy may well broaden access to care by moving more clients through the system, managed care organizations have little incentive to seek out difficult clients (Hawthorn and Hough 1997) or to provide for the extensive needs and long-term social supports required by individuals with chronic conditions (Bazelon Center 1995: 9).

Providers at Venture were concerned about the needs of their clients with long-term or chronic illnesses. According to one case manager, "You are limited in time; we have had clients who had therapy for fifteen years and never got any better. Now the goal is to get them to end therapy." Consequently, providers found they had to focus on "dealing with specific issues—rather than long-term needs and problems." Providers at Venture also found that a reliance on medication had replaced their traditional emphasis on psychotherapy and psychosocial development. During the focus group interview one therapist flatly stated, "Medication is it, there is stabilization of symptoms with very little thought of what someone needs beyond that." The providers concurred that managed care was not going to meet the needs of those with chronic mental illnesses, and that more people "would end up in the criminal justice system." One MSW in private practice whom I interviewed informed me that a managed care case manager had told her to

> tell the patient, convince her to go on medication because we think it will solve her problems quicker. They want to do whatever to get the patient, not better, but in shape and shipped out, off their books.

Another consequence of managed care is the use of fewer providers, and the reliance on providers who offer mental health care with the lowest cost. According to one managed care representative, the "marketplace will use the discipline with the lowest cost;" where data on efficacy is scarce (as in mental health) "there is a built-in tendency to assume equal efficacy and therefore go to the lowest cost provider" (Schreter et al. 1994: 105). Practically, this means use of providers with less specialized training (master's level clinicians and social workers rather than PhD psychologists and psychiatrists). The primary role of the psychiatrist will be to prescribe medication (Luhrmann 2000). Psychologists are treated even more harshly in the managed care environment; one managed care representative views "psychotherapy as the only field of health where the patient receives the treatment the therapist is trained to provide, rather than the treatment the patient's condition requires" (Schreter et al. 1994: 120). All of the PhD psychologists I interviewed described difficulty getting on certain managed care panels "because they don't want a PhD psychologist." Some providers report that they no longer list psychotherapy as a specialty since managed care companies have little interest in reimbursing this form of treatment (Alperin 1997).

Other professionals have redefined psychotherapy to fit into a managed care environment (Austad and Hoyt 1992; Hoyt and Austad 1992) by developing treatment modalities that are short-term, eclectic, and effective, those that are "time-sensitive, focused, and oriented toward achieving clearly defined goals" (Ludwig and Moltz 1997: 260). Much of this short-term, focused therapy is most effectively performed by social workers who have had their employment opportunities expand in the managed care marketplace. Master's level clinicians are also most likely to serve as cost-containment case managers and to fill other types of administrative roles in managed care companies (Schreter et al. 1994), and the curriculum of many MSW programs is changing accordingly.

THE ETHICAL CHALLENGE OF MANAGED CARE

A growing body of literature discusses the ethical dilemmas faced by health care providers under managed care (for example, Bondeson and Jones 2002; Gervais et al. 1999; Anderlik 2001) and much of it concerns those dilemmas faced specifically by mental health care providers (Fletcher 1998; Galambos 1999; Kirschner and Lachicotte 2001; Ware et al. 2000). Galambos (1999) juxtaposes the tenets of good social work practice that emphasize client need, to cost-containment strategies, which reduce consumer choice and place the provider in the role of a gatekeeper. Furman (2003) also describes the disparate values that differentiate social work and managed mental health care. Turney and Conway (2000) studied six managed health care plans and document ethical concerns with confidentiality as well as clients' rights to services and self-determination. In their ethnographic study of a community mental health center, Kirschner and Lachiocotte (2001) found that providers had a sense of moral outrage and felt threatened by managed care. Ware et al. (2000) reported that these same providers feared deprofessionalization and saw the potential for quality care to deteriorate. All of these concerns were raised by the private practice providers I interviewed.

In addition to concern over access and the quality of care provided by managed care, providers fear that managed care will reduce the quality of the provider-client relationship (Backlar 1996). They are no longer able to serve primarily as advocates for their clients by offering any available treatment that they deem to be beneficial. Instead, they are limited to those treatments that can produce measurable client outcomes and that are cost effective. Managed care subjects the treatment decisions of providers and the provider-client relationship to increased managerial, financial, and bureaucratic scrutiny. Both the quality and quantity of interaction between provider and client may be reduced; providers may have fewer incentives or rewards for exemplary care, and an emphasis on accountability interferes with the therapeutic relationship. As described by Edwards (1997: 200, 211):

> The two most basic components of an analytic therapeutic process, the patient's ability to speak freely and the therapist's capacity to listen freely, are being seriously compromised. . . . I was further distressed with the new form that had recently been adopted by the company. It provided even less opportunity to convey the uniqueness of each person than the previous one. One had the choice of describing a patient, for example, as disheveled, bizarre, inappropriately groomed, or well groomed. None of these categories describe (x).

One of the MSW providers I interviewed became increasingly angry as she described her experience with managed care.

My experience with managed care was very negative. I think it's totally un-
ethical, I think it's totally coercive. One of the things I don't like about managed care is they want you to work for them. You know, they tell me, "Tell
her it's in her best interests, and tell her . . ." It's like, I don't work for you,
and that's not what I believe and I'm not going to tell my patient that. They
coerce mental health professionals as well as patients . . . If you want to stay
on their panel, you have to play their game.

Concerns over the therapeutic process are often described in terms of
the kinds of ethical dilemmas that result when managed care entities implement various forms of oversight review to "manage" the care providers offer. Requests for mental health care are more likely than physical
health care to be denied (Mechanic and McAlpine 1999). Utilization review
and the development of protocols to standardize treatment directly challenge professional authority and expertise (Schlesinger et al. 1997; Shore
and Beigel 1996). Birne-Stone et al. (1997) provide a summary of the questions addressed by most review processes. First, is the treatment medically
necessary? In order to meet the standard of medical necessity the patient
must have a DSM Axis I diagnosis. Second, the treatment must be consistent with national standards. There is the further expectation that the client
will get better with treatment, and that providers establish clear, measurable, and realistic goals. Finally, the treatment plan submitted by the provider must be time- and cost-sensitive.

The following account is from an MSW who had requested more sessions for a client whom she had been seeing long-term who had experienced childhood sexual abuse from her father.

I told the reviewer, "There is no way I can wind this up in a couple months . . .
that's not appropriate treatment." And they said, "You don't understand,
you've been seeing her for a long time, and we need to move along." I told
them, "Do you think you could just get over it if you had been f—-ed by your
father your whole life?"

It is obvious that professional values are undermined by the reliance on
entrepreneurial standards to determine whether treatment should be
made available to a client. In their 1992 survey of utilization review organizations, Schlesinger et al. (1997) found that the greatest number (40 percent) did preserve clinical autonomy, though 14 percent sought to
transform clinical practice by standardizing treatments. Another 25 percent emphasized the establishment of a scientific ethos in developing treatment guidelines. Yet it is likely that "cost-containment and market
mechanisms may increasingly set limits" to job control and decision-making authority," as well as to providers' ability to determine treatment and
wider organizational goals (Soderfeldt et al. 1996: 1222). One psychiatrist
reported that "such experiences contribute to increasing feelings of impo-

tence, disenchantment with our profession, and ultimately to burnout" (Schreter et al. 1994: 112). The loss of autonomy will not only produce higher levels of job dissatisfaction and burnout, it may also have an effect on client outcomes as well by reducing standards for care (Phillips 1997). Aiken and Sloan (1997) found that autonomy and opportunities for authority experienced by nurses on specialized AIDS units were linked to better patient outcomes.

Managed care at Venture produced more bureaucratic rules and paperwork, which providers found frustrating. However, treatment decisions were still made by professionals and were reviewed only if they exceeded the maximum number of outpatient visits. Since the agency is a nonprofit organization with strong institutional links to clinical training and research, the bottom line is still defined by professional standards. This is exemplified by the fact that Venture had not restricted its formulary in response to limited resources, and encouraged providers to utilize the newer, more effective (and expensive) psychotropic medications. Such reliance on more sophisticated medications is directly related to a provider's sense of upholding professionally defined treatment standards.

The providers in private practice I interviewed all found that managed care had introduced more paperwork into their practices, with comments such as the "excessive documentation was not necessary, it takes time away from my work with clients, with continuing my education, my own self-care. I have to wear too many work hats." The paperwork associated with managed care was also cited by survey respondents as a significant source of stress.

As described earlier, in managed care organizations decisions to reimburse mental health services are based upon external determinations of "medical necessity." Only if a client's given mental health condition meets DSM criteria, results in impaired social functioning, and treatment is effective and justified by the professional literature and can be monitored for effectiveness, will it meet the condition of medical necessity (Moffic 1997). This is a very difficult standard to apply in mental health care since there is little consensus on what constitutes appropriate care (Clark et al. 1994), as illustrated by the experience of an MSW whom I interviewed:

> I gave her a diagnosis of adjustment disorder, and the reviewer said, "What are her symptoms?" And he said, "It doesn't sound like adjustment disorder to me. It sounds like she is pretty normal." And I had to sit there and tell the client that her services would not be covered because the insurance company didn't think she was sick.

If one views mental health as a continuum, then more mental health is better and meeting the condition of medical necessity invariably means doing less for the client (Herron 1997). By adhering to a strict medical model of care, managed care companies avoid providing reimbursement for what they perceive as "problems in living" (Schreter et al. 1994: 52). In describing a newly hired chief utilization reviewer's approach to treatment decisions, Moffic (1997: 162) found that utilization review based upon a strict standard of medical necessity had the anticipated result that

> there would be no long-term psychotherapy for panic disorders, as obviously medication should do the trick. Children with conduct disorders would not be authorized for hospitalization for their parent's convenience. For suicidal depressed patients, three inpatient days and you better be out . . . and of course, no psychoanalysis would be authorized, even if it was provided at a low fee that would fit under the benefit plans.

Three types of patients are most at risk for having treatment denied under managed care systems (Moffic 1997): First, individuals who are likely to show some kind of spontaneous improvement without treatment, including individuals who experience acute episodes of depression due to some stressful life event such as divorce or death. Second, individuals who are not likely to exhibit any improvement regardless of the treatment offered, which would include many individuals with schizophrenia. Third, individuals who are at risk for some kind of negative treatment response (for example, those with masochistic or narcissistic personality traits). A strident definition of medical necessity will result in dramatically lower levels of overall mental health and functioning. Managed care companies also prefer clients who display "readiness," who are compliant with recommended treatments and are willing to openly discuss their problems. Once again, those with more severe illness (especially schizophrenia) are not likely to exhibit treatment readiness.

In addition, managed care has raised serious questions about client confidentiality. Moffic (1997: 97) notes that managed care entities ask for more information than any other third-party purchaser. They ask for copies of notes providers keep on patients, perform site visits to review medical records, and may even interview patients to verify treatment. Such actions are motivated by a bureaucratic distrust of clinicians, and can result in patient distrust of the clinician as well. High-tech management information systems allow financial managers to track client outcomes as well as to arrive at precise provider-based costs of care summaries, and represent a viable threat to client confidentiality. Such threats were cited by almost all of the providers I interviewed, and one MSW gave as an example her dilemma of needing to protect a client's confidentiality while trying to get authorization for care.

> A client will ask me, can't you just fill this form out and not let them know I'm impotent, or my partner is same sex. So I just don't give that information, but then the company says, "This is very vague . . . What is going on here?"

> I say, "Sorry, I'm not at liberty to say, the client has asked me not to." I can say this is true, and these are some of the symptoms, and this is what they need. And I resent having to negotiate with a managed care company about stuff like that.

Despite the constraints of various types of oversight review, providers are bound by professional norms to act as advocates for their clients, and are ultimately held accountable for treatment practices. Thus providers are legally bound to appeal decisions by utilization reviewers that could result in harm to the patient (for example, denying hospitalization for a client whom the provider feels will attempt suicide). The provider is also in the position of having to inform the client about how the system works, even though providers can also be dropped from networks if they disclose such information in a disparaging manner. Tuttle and Woods (1997: 52) list "disparagement of the managed care firm" as the second-most common reason providers are dropped from mental health panels, the most common reason being inappropriate relationships with clients. One MSW recounted her experience after telling a client the provider would be penalized for requesting more sessions, and the client complained directly to the insurance company.

> I got reprimanded, and the reprimand contained a veiled threat that I could be sued for breach of contract, and I felt like a prostitute, and it was at that point that I wrote a letter of resignation to that company, and it felt great.

This provider went on to drop out of other panels that were "a pain in the neck" and was considering canceling the rest of her contracts "and being out of managed care entirely."

The most notable ethical dilemma arises when the provider receives some kind of financial incentive for limiting patient care, whether in the form of capitated payments or case rates, retainers for seeing a fixed number of clients, or progressively decreasing reimbursement to clinicians for longer courses of treatment (Lazarus and Pollock 1997). If cost savings are directed back to client care (as in nonprofit or public systems of care) the ethical dilemma of reduced care is diminished; it is enhanced in profit-based systems. Providers in this situation face the very real concern that they may lose their jobs as a result of their treatment decisions (Backlar 1996); if their costs are viewed as too high they may be dropped from panels, or else be let go from public agencies.

Ultimately these ethical dilemmas reflect substantial conflict over professionally based standards of care and standards based upon a more technically driven business ethic motivated primarily by fiscal savings or profit. Providers face a direct challenge to their professional prerogative to determine what kind of care is most suitable for a given client. There are two critical variables that will determine the overall effect managed care will have upon the autonomy and authority of providers. First, how much involvement do providers have in the development and implementation of new managed care guidelines and clinical standards? Second, what standards are decisions of care being made upon? Is the determinant factor cost, or quality care (including access)? If providers have a direct financial stake, they will be more likely to emphasize cost savings than access or quality care. Furthermore, there is an obvious conflict between providing the full continuum of care needed by the chronic, or long-term, client and a system designed to provide as little care as possible.

CONCLUSION

Mental health care, in response to efficiency demands made by its environment, has indeed changed in response to "the viscidities of the market" (Meyer 1990: 211). Yet both Meyer (1990) and Heydeband (1990) view the new commodification and its concomitant technocratic rationality as unstable because of the inherent conflict between opposing forms of rationality and value orientation. In mental health care these conflicts are evidenced in debates over cost versus quality and access, short-term versus long-term therapy, cure versus prevention and intervention and the series of ethical dilemmas faced by providers. The next chapters examine the effect of managed care on the work experiences of providers in the public sector.

NOTES

1. There is some overlap in my use of the model of community-based care and Light's (1997) ideal type, but the terms are not equivalent. The community-based care model I am referring to combines elements of both the community and professionally based systems, and refers to a specific ideological orientation to the treatment of mental health care problems.

2. The problem of who does this research and the standards by which it is evaluated are set is an important one for future research.

5   The Padded Cell

Bureaucracy and Control over Provider's Work

If you ever saw the guy on the Ed Sullivan show—the one with all the plates, and he had to make sure all the plates rotate at the same time; that's what my job is like. I'm the plate guy. (MSW in public sector)

Sociologists have long been fascinated with the consequences of bureaucracy (dehumanization, trained incapacity) as well as with the conflict between bureaucratic and professional authority, and with the degree of control and autonomy individuals have in bureaucratic settings. Bureaucracy is an important form of social control, and, as Weber (1946) predicted, it is a form of organization that has become inescapable in modern society. Managed care rationalizes caregiving and emphasizes efficiency and cost-containment. It imposes a rational business ethic and corresponding system of bureaucratic control on organizations that had previously operated in terms of a professionally based moral foundation. Consequently, managed care poses a threat to the professional autonomy and decision-making power of providers. In this chapter I use both qualitative and quantitative data to analyze the organizational contexts within which providers work. In order to analyze care within a bureaucracy, I focus on providers working in public, community-based mental health systems.

ORGANIZATION OF MENTAL HEALTH CARE

Most clients receive mental health care as outpatients rather than inpatients; furthermore, the majority of this care is provided by multiservice mental health care organizations (referred to as MHOs).[1] The MHO provides a broad array of services to diverse client populations; the "worried well," individuals with severe persistent mental illnesses, individuals with developmental disabilities, and individuals with substance abuse prob-

83

lems. MHOs may also provide services to children and adolescents as well as adults. The services that are provided and the clients who are served reflect wider social values and priorities, and these have undergone a series of shifts from institutionalization, to community-based, to managed care. Because MHOs operate in turbulent institutional environments, they experience "cyclical legitimacy crises" (Hasenfeld 1992: 1), since organizational form changes more slowly than do institutional demands. For example, only recently has the institutional environment begun to demand greater mental health services for children; it will take MHOs some time to develop the organizational structures to provide these services. In the meantime, MHOs will be subject to criticism for not providing adequate care to children.

Given the diversity of services and client populations, MHOs are difficult to characterize. Researchers have described them as unrewarding places to work, both because of the clients and because of the bureaucratic context. Clients with severe mental illness provide little positive feedback and have been labeled as "undesirable" (Atwood 1982; Lang 1981; Stern and Minkoff 1979). Furthermore, the majority of these clients do not need therapy, but case management and supportive services (Mechanic 1986; Harris and Bergman 1987). Case management may not be deemed as professionally challenging or rewarding as therapy.

Furthermore, MHOs have generally operated in the public domain. Historically, the public mental health system has served as a safety net for those clients who are poorer, more disabled, and less desirable (Institute of Medicine 1997; Frank et al. 1997). Public MHOs are funded by a diverse mix of federal, state, and county funds with most clients receiving some form of Medicare, or Medicaid. Consequently, resources are limited and providers are likely to be dissatisfied with opportunities for salary gains and promotion. Oberlander (1990), in a survey of 601 mental health care providers, found that staff working with the seriously mentally ill were more vulnerable to both stress and dissatisfaction with their work. Ben-Dror (1994) reported that low pay, followed by feelings of stress and a lack of participation in decisions about clients, were the major reasons employees left community mental health residential services.

On a more theoretical level, MHOs have been characterized as having contradictory and ambiguous objectives, loose-coupling of formal structure (work roles) and technical activities (the work performed) from client outcomes, and informal systems of organizational control and authority (Hasenfeld 1992; Scheid-Cook 1990, 1991). Because MHOs contain both professional and bureaucratic occupational groups, they are sites for conflict to emerge between the experts and the bureaucrat (Scott 1985). Professionals in mental health organizations have less authority within their organization than other groups of health care professionals (Scott and

Lammers 1985; Scott 1983). This is because there is a dearth of solutions or proven technologies to aid providers in their work (Mechanic 1986, 1994; Rochefort 1989).[2] This is in part why MHOs have ambiguous and contradictory goals. In addition, many of the professionals in mental health organizations are professionals "in transition," seeking greater recognition; this is especially true of nurses and social workers (Guy 1985) although other types of mental health workers (rehabilitation and substance abuse counselors) seek greater professional recognition for their work as well.

MHOs are also structurally diverse; they vary in size from a single agency that provides all the necessary (or available) services to a community, to a consortium of different agencies performing specialized functions (Wagenfeld and Robin 1976). There is also a wide range of work roles and services provided, and, as has been found in other human service organizations (Glisson and Durick 1988), there is likely to be variation in job characteristics even when similar tasks are performed. In addition, mental health care is provided by a number of different types of professionals: psychiatrists, psychologists, social workers, and nurses (Scott and Lammers 1985). Consequently, there is much potential for interprofessional conflict.

Because of their professional diversity, MHOs are excellent sites for the study of different "segments," those occupational groups where members share common work activities, values, and identities (Halpern 1992). Different segments may correspond to occupational or professional subcultures; different occupations within an organization give rise to multiple cultures (Gregory 1983; Meyerson 1991). One primary source of group identity is professional background, members of a profession share a common approach to their clients by virtue of their education. In addition to professional orientations, providers are also subject to the demands of their organizational work role. For example, case managers may be nurses, social workers, therapists, or rehabilitation counselors. Case managers with RN licenses are professional nurses, yet their job is to manage cases. Similarly, MSWs are considered to be professional social workers, yet if they manage cases, their occupation is that of case manager. While professional orientations and training may vary, those performing case management are likely to face similar problems and have common experiences, leading to the formation of an occupational identity, which may then result in professional certification. Consequently, it is important to distinguish between professional and occupational (or work role) segments. Understanding the experiences of providers performing different work roles is critical because different segments will seek to protect their treatment domains with impending resource restrictions and rationing of services (Hafferty and Light 1995).

BUREAUCRATIC CONTROL, PROFESSIONAL STATUS AND CONFLICT

Central to professional status is autonomy and control over one's work. Summarizing the various definitions of "professional" Hafferty and Wolinsky (1991) identify three characteristics of professionalism: monopolization of knowledge (i.e., expert identification), autonomy in work performance, and authority over clients. Central to legitimacy as a "professional" is licensure and the authority and control over one's work (Freidson 1984).

It is important to clarify the meanings of control, authority, and autonomy. Soderfeldt et al. (1996) distinguish between skill discretion (control over one's work) and decision authority (freedom to make decisions about one's work). Skill discretion involves task discretion, routinization, and opportunities to learn new things. Skill discretion is analogous to decision latitude, which has received much attention by Karasek and his associates (Karasek and Theorell 1990). Decision authority refers to how much input individuals have into organizational policies and decisions, and whether they have authority over the work of others. Consequently, authority reflects the degree of power individuals have relative to others, whereas skill discretion refers to how much authority they have over their own work. As noted earlier, mental health care providers may have greater skill discretion (due to uncertain treatment technologies) and less authority relative to other groups of health care providers.

Autonomy also entails the degree to which one is free from close supervisory attention (Schwalbe 1986), or is able to make decisions without fear of organizational intervention. Consequently autonomy will encompass both skill discretion and authority. Professionals are granted high degrees of autonomy by virtue of their expert status; they can make decisions about their work without relying on the approval of others in the organization. Generally, the more control exerted by the organization over the work of its employees, the less control, authority, and autonomy the individual will have. Because of the uncertain technology in mental health, providers often have assumed a good deal of power (skill discretion) over how they do their work (Cook and Wright 1995), even without a great deal of professional recognition, though this situation may well change with managed care. Yet because providers work in public bureaucracies, they may find they have less input into organizational policies and procedures (decision authority) and supervisors may reduce their degree of autonomy.[3]

MHO psychiatrists and psychologists are the ultimate "legitimate" professionals, wielding considerable power and authority. Yet the majority of care is provided by nurses and social workers; both groups have traditionally sought greater professional recognition, power, and autonomy.

The internal differentiation between nurses and social workers constitutes a threat to their professional status, as does the fact that both occupations are dominated by women (Hall 1986). Further, the ideology of care and commitment to others may be inconsistent with professional domination of expert, technical knowledge (Trice 1993). With higher professional status, providers are in a better position to challenge organizational (or bureaucratic) forms of control. The central issue is whether work is guided by standardized rules and formal procedures, or whether the provider has a wide degree of skill discretion, decision latitude, and autonomy.

Sociologists studying health care organizations have described the potential conflict between bureaucratic and professional control (Scott 1981, 1992). Organizations rely upon external controls, formal rules, and direct supervision while professionals rely upon internalized codes of conduct learned via professionalization socialization. Regulation of professional activity occurs by means of admission criteria, education, socialization, licensure, professional associations, and examining boards that are generally composed of one's peers (Moore 1970). Such mechanisms of professional control run counter to the principles of organized bureaucracies (Larson 1977).

However, the relationship between professional and bureaucratic authority is complex and conflict is not always evident, nor necessary. Scott (1992) distinguishes between heteronomous professional organizations, where professionals are subordinate to administrative authority, and autonomous professional organizations, where professionals have considerable power and authority. In autonomous professional organizations, bureaucratic positions of organizational control are likely to be held by members of the profession. Yet researchers have generally found evidence of conflict between professional and bureaucratic authority in professional organizations (Hall 1986). This is because bureaucratic decision-making is hierarchical, rule-governed, and based upon individual accountability (Waters 1989). Professional, or collegial, decision-making is egalitarian, consensual, and based upon individual autonomy. Furthermore, the non-routine nature of the work in professional organizations mitigates against centralized, bureaucratic control (Anderson 1992).

Freidson (1984) has argued that formalization rather than deprofessionalization of professional control occurs when an administrative elite of professionals evaluates the performance of "rank and file" professionals. Examples of such mechanisms of formal control are formal review committees and standardized evaluations of work performance. The replacement of internalized professional norms and standards with organizational arrangements that monitor practice is referred to as corporate rationalization (Anderson 1992). Corporate rationalization has the effect of delegitimating the decision-making power of the individual (Scott 1985). As described by Starr (1982), organizational control over the pace and routines of work, as well as the close scrutiny of mistakes, contributes to the loss of professional autonomy of individual doctors. However, since doctors themselves have served as agents of formal control, the profession itself does not become deprofessionalized or proletariatized (Scott 1985; Starr 1982). Yet the decline in the autonomy of the individual professional will result in the loss of a sense of professional community (Freidson 1984). Managed care represents an obvious extension of the logic of corporate rationality, and may also involve some degree of deprofessionalization, depending on the specific mechanisms whereby care is managed and how much input providers have into the management of care.

In the wider health care sector, physicians have become adept managers (Rodwin 1993). While their work is indeed subject to greater bureaucratic oversight in managed care organizations, physicians have been able to maintain control by virtue of their professional expertise (Griffiths and Hughs 1999; Hoff and McCaffrey 1996; Lupton 1997; Weiss and Fitzpatrick, 1997). Decisions about clinical care must rely upon medical expertise. For example, Weiss and Fitzpatrick (1997) found that while physicians in Great Britain conform to principles of cost-containment, clinical autonomy was maintained. Professional logics of care changed to incorporate bureaucratic and corporate principles. However, health care providers with less legitimate claims to expert knowledge have more difficulty maintaining clinical autonomy. Furthermore, where treatment technologies are ambiguous or contradictory (as in mental health) there is an increased likelihood that bureaucratic standards of care will prevail.

MHOs are autonomous professional organizations; supervisors generally have a clinical background, consider themselves professionals, often have a caseload and work on a fairly equal level with other providers. There are also relatively few layers of bureaucratic stratification and authority in MHOs. For example, while CARE is large for an MHO (approximately ninety direct care providers serve over 2,000 clients), there are only three levels of authority: supervisors of individual programs or teams, program administrators (or coordinators), and project directors. Directors and administrators have greater distance from clients, yet still interact frequently (and informally) with staff. Supervisors have caseloads, and work on a fairly egalitarian basis with other providers. This organizational form is also typical of SUPPORT and the twenty-nine MHOs studied in Wisconsin (Scheid and Greenley 1997).

Despite the relatively few layers of management (low complexity) and professional orientation of mental health care administrators, many MHOs still have a bureaucratic ethos. Drolen (1990) reported that directors of MHOs were more concerned with control and efficiency than creativity or innovation, despite the fact that Gowdy and Rapp (1989) found effective MHOs were those with a "can-do" (i.e., innovative and creative) attitude. Therefore, there is still potential for conflict in MHOs between bureaucratic and professional authorities, and providers may well face threats to their professional status. In a study of a counseling organization, Nijsmans (1991) found that professional imperatives were more powerful than organizational rules, which were often seen as incompatible with professional ideologies.

In MHOs, interprofessional conflicts constitute another threat to professional status. Interprofessional conflict is often characterized by jurisdictional disputes (Abbott 1988) over treatment ideologies, which services to provide, or how best to achieve organizational (treatment) objectives. Psychiatrists and nurses may emphasize the central role of medication, while social workers may stress rehabilitation and skills training. Because MHOs serve different client groups, and offer diverse services, they have a wide variety of professional and occupational (work role) segments, which are likely to disagree with each other over treatment and service provision. Shared organizational positions (i.e., shift or unit) can also lead to similar perceptions and treatment preferences (Doherty and Harry 1976). The organization's structure of authority is critical to resolution of these disputes. It provides an arena in which disagreements can be resolved collegially, and maintain a provider's sense of autonomy; or it may resolve disputes bureaucratically, and limit the provider's autonomy. Autonomy and a sense of control over one's work, as well as input into organizational decisions, contribute to the provider's sense of self-efficacy and self-esteem, and can have a critical impact on their level of job satisfaction as well as the quality of care they provide.

MENTAL HEALTH WORK

It is important to have some understanding of the work that providers do: what their day is like and how they perceive the organization around them and professional interactions. I will therefore begin with data from my in-depth interviews with providers who worked in CARE and SUPPORT. Two case managers (one at CARE and one at SUPPORT) used the metaphor of the plate guy to describe their work: "I feel like the person on the stage with a stick holding up a stack of plates while on roller skates." In other words, providers "have to wear a lot of different hats." The mental health centers where I conducted my fieldwork are extremely busy places. Clients fill available space, and providers are constantly on the go. The phones ring incessantly. Caseloads at CARE were thirty to thirty-five clients; SUPPORT's were a little fewer; both are high for intensive case management with severely mentally disabled clients. In addition to direct client care, providers must fit team meetings, staff meetings, meetings with clients' families, and running around the community into a typical day. "I do a bunch of different stuff, arts and crafts, verbal groups, lots of independent living skills stuff, budgeting, going out into the community, into client's houses," reports a female vocational education counselor. Complicating the "typical" day are the constant, ongoing crises with clients, including suicides, emergency hospitalizations, arrests, and cases of abuse or drug overdose. Following are some descriptions of a "typical" day, to give a sense of what mental health work entails:

> Working in this kind of program, you do anything and everything: paperwork, documentation, representing the program. Assisting with supervision to cooking, helping someone to get dry clothes, holding someone who is crying, running groups, driving the van. A lot depends on the needs of my clients; I do a lot of phone work, talking to agencies, making referrals, talking with families. I work a long day: 7:30 to 5:30. (Female case manager)

One of the difficulties of the job is coordinating client care with members of the treatment team.

> We have a meeting in the morning and go over our tickler cards and decide what we are doing that day. A tickler card is a 5 x 8 card we keep for each client, and we keep a list of contacts and how many times you need to see them (depending on their level of functioning and treatment plan). And that day is all in the appointment book: who has appointments, who needs injections, whether I need a car. I don't go out every day, but I like to get out and see the clients. There is a lot of freedom to decide how to schedule our days; it doesn't always work out that way, but it is a nice part of the job. (Female case manager)

Flexibility allows providers to feel a sense of control and empowerment: "It's really nice as you have total autonomy, you can figure out who you are going to see." Many providers left other types of mental health work (especially institutional care) because they liked the independence and freedom of "smaller, more independent" community-based programs. The lack of hierarchical structure was consistently cited as one of the major benefits of community-based mental health work. Providers were critical of organizational structures that did not provide them with flexibility, or involvement in decisions.

> I'd like to have more involvement in decisions that are made about the program. I'd like to have more flexibility about my time, so I can arrange some kind of schedule to do paperwork without having to worry about other things. (Male case manager)

Despite the fact that community MHOs did provider greater flexibility and input than other types of mental health organizations (especially inpatient units), there was considerable evidence of bureaucratic control, as well as conflict with professional standards. Criticism of the organization generally focused on the lack of involvement in decisions, or on supervisors who were "too rigid." Good supervisors were those who were supportive and allowed the staff to do what they thought best for a client. The best supervisors were those who worked closely with their staff, and who also maintained a caseload, though this made the supervisor's job very complicated. One supervisor described her job in the following way:

> I begin with scheduling to make sure all areas are covered, make sure charts are in order, quality assurance is involved. I go to lots of meetings, staff meeting every morning, and again in the afternoon, plus staffing with doctors. Plus we do groups; I am a working supervisor, I have a caseload of eight clients. I have mixed feelings about being a supervisor, I always consider the staff's feelings, how they will respond to a situation. I try to make sure they understand it has to be done, I won't ask anything of them I wouldn't do myself. There is a lot of autonomy, mutual respect here. Treatment plans reflect mutual input.

Another supervisor also stressed the need for "interactive management" where everyone has "input." This supervisor also described the potential conflict between administrative and clinical work.

> Yes, I do have a caseload, fourteen clients, which is more than the other supervisors. I do good case management, but if I have a meeting at the area office and I have a crisis with a client, I'll cancel the meeting. But if it's just visiting with the client, and a meeting is called, it's hard to know which is best.

Before examining bureaucratic and professional conflict directly, it is important to consider the provider's sense of accomplishment as mental health professionals, and their feelings about their professional status. The typical duties of a case manager do not generally require a high degree of technical expertise, and this was a problem for some providers: "I think anybody could be doing this, it does not take a master's degree." Providers wanted their job titles to reflect their professional qualifications and abilities. They were aware that they served as a safety net in the wider mental health sector, especially when faced with the persistent resource shortages characteristic of public mental health. "The message is we're public, we're psychiatric clients, we don't count."

Despite this acknowledgment of status differentials, all of the providers I interviewed loved their work.

> When I saw myself in this field, I had a picture of myself with a master's or doctorate, sitting in some nice office and doing counseling. But I love going out like a social worker and seeing the neighborhoods, the family, and knowing the client at home. (Female MSW case manager)

One MSW who left private practice stated simply: "I got tired of the inside of my office." Another provider argued that the job of case manager took more skills and expertise than those required by counseling or therapy.

> That's the whole notion of what therapy is, that's where the big bucks are, and that's professional. And just running around the way we do, that's something that's not all that difficult, one that you need special skills for. But I guess it doesn't bother me that much. I think this job takes more skills than any therapist, and it's much more difficult than what the psychiatrists do. We are the mediators; we do the really hard work, we spend time with these folks. (Male MSW case manager)

These quotes exemplify how providers resolve some of the contradictions between managing care and providing care discussed in Chapter 2. Providers also had a great deal of control over their work; case managers were out of the office much of the time and had a great deal of latitude in how they organized their day and met the needs of their clients. When asked in written questionnaires how much control they had over their jobs, close to one-half of providers at both CARE and SUPPORT responded with "a great deal" (43.9 percent and 45.8 percent, respectively), and over one-third reported "some control" (43.9 percent and 37.5 percent, respectively). Providers at both CARE and SUPPORT also reported extremely high levels of satisfaction with their job and careers.

When asked to explore sources of stress and other aspects about their jobs they disliked, providers at both sites focused on paperwork, bureaucratic demands, and conflicts with administrative authorities. Paperwork was especially a problem at CARE; over 55 percent of the providers cited paperwork as that which they most disliked about their jobs (compared to only 25 percent of providers at SUPPORT citing paperwork). This may be due to the larger caseloads at CARE, or the fact that CARE had a more bureaucratized system of client tracking, in part due to an external grant. It may also reflect the fact that SUPPORT was a decentralized system, whereas CARE was more centralized.

However, providers at both MHOs found bureaucratic demands to be a considerable source of frustration and stress. Sometimes the source of bureaucratic demands was "the county bureaucracy which interferes with good management and care of clients." At other times providers were frustrated with "trying to negotiate the system" and diverse sets of rules and standards. The layers of bureaucracy and interactions with other agencies created a flood of paperwork; almost all of the providers interviewed described how overwhelmed they were by the amount of paperwork they had to complete.

> Going home year after year not being able to complete all work required despite working overtime, weekends, and holidays. It is very disheartening to

always have more work at the end of the day than you started with. (Female case manager)

More often than the county bureaucracy, the targeted source of frustration were upper-level administrators who make "decisions about how things will go without knowing how things are." Generally it was the team supervisor who most undermined the professional status of providers:

My supervisor openly criticizes and ridicules team members in front of others. I am stressed when there is too much work to do, and unrealistic expectations placed upon me by my supervisor . . . when supervisors make poorly informed decisions. (Female case manager)

Providers also mentioned not feeling appreciated, or lacking involvement in decisions as common sources of stress and dissatisfaction. As one provider stated, "It would help to have some validation of our efforts." Inadequate support or the feeling of not accomplishing what one wanted to because of bureaucratic interference were also mentioned as sources of burnout. This will be discussed in the next chapter.

Clients with severe mental illness are needy, and often their needs cannot wait for a monthly appointment. Coordination and communication are central to providing the type of integrated care needed for clients. Multidisciplinary treatment teams are now the standard approach; the team consists of different professionals who provide the care needed by the client. When I conducted my fieldwork, both CARE and SUPPORT were first developing treatment teams, and providers spoke highly of the multidisciplinary team and interprofessional relations. Treatment teams were universally viewed as necessary to the provider's own sense of fulfillment and satisfaction, as well as good client care: "The only reason anyone survives is that you work as a team; if it becomes totally overwhelming somebody is always there to say, I'll pick this up for you."

However, this kind of support can also lead to conflict. In a multidisciplinary treatment team, providers must learn to work together on a daily basis and to make collaborative decisions about client care. Communication between providers and programs becomes central. Case managers must deal with providers who work in the different specialized programs for medication, vocational rehabilitation, or skills training that are needed by clients.

Communication is the biggest thing, because you have people from different disciplines coming from different backgrounds, and everyone has their own view; its hard to ensure that everyone is coming from the same mindset. We do well, and we provide integrated care, but communication from one part to another is sometimes lacking. We need the separate entities, but we need to ensure communication is more uniform so that people understand the reason behind a policy. (Male MSW case manager)

The major communication problems arose between providers in the different programs that provided services to clients (supported employment, medication clinic, occupational therapy, crisis stabilization). Providers in these more specialized units often reported conflict with case managers, and case managers also complained that they were not informed of changes in their clients' condition or care. The issue of responsibility for client care reflects jurisdictional disputes. As one occupational therapist said, "Case managers can only do so much, clients need occupational therapy, day programs, medication counseling." Another provider at a day program described the jurisdictional dispute with case managers in the following terms:

> We'd like more contact with the doctors, rather than having to go through the case managers; there are things we notice here that case managers don't see. It's very hard to get up with the case managers. I'm not saying case managers don't care, but sometimes I wonder. (Female provider in clubhouse)

Nurses also spoke of jurisdictional disputes, noting that they could provide more integrated care by meeting the client's medical as well as their psychosocial needs. One nurse stated that "nurses made better case managers than social workers." On the other hand, social workers were critical of the dominance of medical professionals over a client's medication needs:

> I rely on others to give me feedback about clients. I try to work with the doctors to involve me in decisions, especially about medications. For example, they changed the meds on one of my clients—which then led to bizarre behavior. It went on for a month before they let us know what was going on. (Female MSW case manager)

However, the majority of providers were very enthusiastic about their relationships with their colleagues. The best interprofessional relations occurred when providers were "all coming from the same direction, then there is a lot of support and support giving." Yet this is not always the case. One supervisor described his team as a "vocal group of people, and there are different ways to get to the same goal and people are willing to express their ideas, and other people respect that." The critical variable seemed to be the degree of mutual respect, and respect for divergent views, that providers granted each other. "People here are good—we are understanding of each other and know the problems we face." When providers talked about instances of interprofessional conflict, they talked about working in places where "politically, philosophically, I didn't feel like I fit with most of those folks; I crashed heads with a lot of people." Often this conflict was over treatment ideology: "We are much more person-centered, at X they were much more medically oriented." Or: "They treated clients very poorly, very authoritarian." Sometimes the sense of "cooperation and acceptance" failed.

> Sometimes I don't like working with other staff members. There's one person I don't agree with, and he's disrespectful, and he doesn't see that. He wants me to agree with everything he does, and he fights back. I mean, we can barely agree to disagree. It's really hard when we are working with the same client. (Female nurse case manager)

This situation was atypical; while providers experienced confrontations and disagreements over appropriate treatment actions, they "agreed with [each other's] right to choose how they wanted to work with a client." In other words, most providers protected each other's authority and autonomy, even though this could be difficult.

> The stress for me is I have to keep in mind how it (my decisions about a client) impact on other people, and keep from getting wrapped up in this is good for this person. (Male MSW case manager)

Thus autonomy is important in provider's work. Organizations are critical to the sense of accomplishment and satisfaction necessary for effective mental health work. While the mental health programs in which the providers I interviewed had organizational policies, "the policies still allow us our autonomy—you don't feel your hands are tied in deciding how to deal with a client." That is, providers had a great deal of skill discretion and autonomy. However, I have described the experiences of providers before the advent of managed care. In the following section, I turn to a consideration of how the work of providers at CARE has changed with managed care.

A PUBLIC SECTOR MANAGED CARE SYSTEM

CARE has been developing a managed care model of service delivery in which the organization serves as both a manager and a provider of care. The administrators at CARE responded to wider institutional demands for managed care, and developed their own managed care plan before the state mandated managed care. Part of their concern was that state-mandated managed care would result in the state's selecting a managed care organization to manage care for all public sector programs, and administrators at CARE felt that they would not be able to maintain their system of care under external control. In 1996, the system began a very deliberate process of organizational change. As of this writing, it is fully operational as a managed care entity and the various components of managed care have been slowly put into place.

The specific objectives of CARE's managed care system include:

1. Improved cost-effectiveness
2. Improved access to services
3. A focus on short-term treatment with long term treatment with long-term service needs justified through utilization review
4. Measurement of costs and outcomes

Mechanisms have been developed to constrain the unnecessary use of services and to insure that the care provided is appropriate, including service authorization, utilization review, contract management, provision of services with measurable outcomes, and financial management of resources. While services are not fully capitated, and Medicaid revenues are drawn on a fee-for-service basis, clinical and business operations are subject to managed care principles (referred to as Care Management). A per diem rate for each service on a client-by-client basis has been established, and service authorization is required each time a provider (both those within CARE as well as those with whom the agency contracts) renders a service.

CARE is both a payor and provider of services. Separate departments provide care, manage care, administer financial resources, and provide oversight review. Services are authorized for payment, and there is a process of utilization review to ensure that all clients receive clinically appropriate services. A separate division analyzes and evaluates service outcomes. A newly developed management information system is in place to provide the needed infrastructure for managed care. However, the computer system has come with a greater than anticipated share of problems and has been a primary reason for delays in the full implementation of managed care, as well as a major source of dissatisfaction among providers who feel they now treat the computer rather than their clients. During a team meeting the computer system was referred to as a "wounded turtle."

In the fall of 1996 CARE took a great deal of time and organizational effort to identify and measure client-level outcomes. Staff attended a series of workshops on outcome assessment and measurement, and the organization then developed a series of performance-based targets for each department in the system. These performance targets specify both client level outcomes as well as the criteria by which the system will evaluate its services (for example, 85 percent of clients in case management will maintain or improve their level of independent functioning each quarter, as measured by change in service-level acuity). Annual assessments are made of these clinical outcomes in order to monitor performance. These annual reports identify barriers, and note areas for improvement as well as introduce new outcome targets. For example, in the fall of 1999 a target for moving clients to lower levels of care (i.e., graduating clients to medication clinic only status) was introduced in order to improve access to case management.

Not only are outcomes evaluated for the entire organization (or division), but data on specific performance targets are evaluated for each treatment team, and can also be assessed for individual providers. One of the goals set by the managed care director at CARE is to standardize treatment decisions so that the same client problem will receive the same kind of service, no matter what provider the client is assigned to: "Treatment will no longer be 'antidotal'—we are seeking consistency in practice . . . right now there is severe variance in the way each provider does treatment . . . inconsistent practices . . . we need to monitor this and establish practice standards." Consequently, clinician profiling is carried out in order to understand what kinds of client outcomes are associated with what kinds of provider practices. Administrators recognized that developing practice standards would take a great deal of time, attitude change, and cultural change, and they were not unequivocal in their support of the development of such practice standards.

The major change in service delivery has been to reorganize the intake procedures to a single port of entry. Previously, every treatment team and program (for example, the clubhouses or partial hospitalization) had its own intake procedures and had the right to refuse any client referred to that unit by another unit or the county hospital. Consequently, there were "a lot of different ways that people came into the system, which limited client's access to the array of service." Intake has been centralized, and specialized intake providers (hired from within the system) conduct a face-to-face interview with every client referred for services and complete a thorough clinical assessment, collect demographic information, evaluate financial support, and develop an initial treatment plan based on state criteria for care. The intake provider assigns clients to the services they are eligible for and for which their care will be reimbursed. Case managers no longer have authority for determining what types of services their clients may receive; instead this will be done by the intake providers. If case managers seek additional services beyond the initial treatment plan, they must obtain authorization (or certification) for such services.

> The case manager has an initial treatment plan they can build upon. A big part of what will change is the whole idea that if you feel someone is in need of service, you have to have something to back that up. (Supervisor)

Initial certification is set for a limited amount of time, and must be reauthorized if the case manager feels a client is in need of additional time in a given program. The hope is that recertification will help move clients

through the continuum of care by forcing providers to think more cre-
atively about how they can utilize natural supports in the community as
well as alternative services.

> Everybody can say these people won't move, and that's part of the problem
> with our thinking . . . they might well be able to move, and we have to be cre-
> ative to think about how we can help them to move . . . People are going to
> have to work a lot harder . . . what we are trying to do is to be sure we keep
> folks at the appropriate level of services, and that's what consumers want; if
> you talk to someone in a group home, chances are they would like to be in
> their own place. So how can you make that happen? That's a key gap we have
> been talking about. (Supervisor)

In order to deal with the new intake procedures, case management was
restructured. Case managers are now defined by levels: Level 1 case managers have higher caseloads but work with clients with less intensive need;
Level 4 case managers have much lower caseloads, but their clients have
more intensive needs (for example, substance abuse). Case managers had
been organized into treatment teams, with some teams having more expertise in dealing with certain types of clients. Some teams had experienced bottlenecks because they had a higher proportion of difficult clients
who showed little evidence of progress; the treatment teams were reorga-
nized to provide for a more even mix of clients and to allow teams to move
clients on through the system. Consequently, when a new client is referred
to case management from the centralized intake unit, the team is expected
to move its highest functioning client to medication clinic-only status.
"They don't have to . . . But if they don't, they will drown" (Supervisor). A
nurse is also assigned to each team to help transfer clients to the medication unit. Administrators felt that the pressure to move clients through the
system could be beneficial. According to one supervisor, "Managed care
will force us to be more realistic in our treatment goals. Right now we make
clients too dependent on us and most of them would be a lot happier if
given the opportunity to handle their own affairs." Administrators also felt
that managed care would force providers to seek out other supports in the
community.

CARE contracts out a good deal of its services to private (external) agencies and providers. Both "internal" and "external" providers are subject to
the same intake procedures and utilization review requirements. Beginning in 1999 all external providers have been subject to extensive review
to ensure that they meet organizational criteria for effective service delivery. I was able to attend meetings of the very large committee (represent-
ing all the major departments within CARE) that performed the service
evaluations, and found the process to be fair, and guided primarily by a
concern that external agencies indeed addressed the client need for which
they sought reimbursement. A performance profile for in-house use has

been developed, which standardizes the criteria for the evaluation of providers. Each agency is discussed at length and with consideration by the review committee. Providers at CARE visited external agencies and gave them ample time to address any weaknesses or concerns before terminating a contract. Terminated contracts are allowed an appeals hearing, and if the contract was still denied, the external provider could appeal directly to the Director of the Area Authority.

In implementing managed care, CARE is consciously seeking to preserve the goals of community-based, integrated care. First, they are seeking to meet the needs of the public sector population eligible for services and hope to make services accessible to the entire population, not just to those with serious mental illnesses. They are seeking to preserve the comprehensive, continuous, integrated system of services developed in the past fifteen years, and to extend and improve that system. A triage system has been developed to offer comprehensive community services and to reduce the use of inpatient care. Finally, CARE is on its way to eliminating the two-tiered system of care by funding private providers to care for public clients and funding public providers to develop services that can compete for private dollars.

Despite the ideological commitment to comprehensive, continuous care, there has been a great deal of conflict over short-term treatment associated with managed care versus longer-term treatment and social supports associated with community-based care. Utilization and concurrent review are housed within the separate managed care division, and members of this team want short-term treatment while the front-line clinical care providers are arguing for longer periods of certification. Administrators are divided: while there is certainly pressure for shorter periods of certification (in order to increase access), they do not want "to overburden clinicians so they spend all their time doing paperwork and seeking recertification." This concern was also cited by the committee evaluating the contracts of the external providers, and points to the potential of managed care to increase organizational inefficiencies due to the proliferation of paperwork.

PRELIMINARY EVALUATION OF MANAGED CARE

The providers I interviewed and who completed questionnaires in 1998 expressed concern that managed care would limit access to services, and that the "over-concern with the cost of care might prohibit clients with severe, persistent mental illnesses from getting the services they needed" (MSW provider). Providers know their clients well, and realize that severe mental illnesses require long-term care and intensive social supports. It is unclear how managed care will meet the needs of their clients:

When we first started hearing about managed care I wondered—how is this going to work with a person who can't hold a job, who needs ongoing services, but they aren't in the hospital? Who is going to pay for that? (Nurse provider)

The data collected in the late spring of 2000 allow for some preliminary assessment of the ability of CARE to provide mental health care that meets both bureaucratic and professional standards of care. The degree of frustration and anger expressed about managed care is striking. While in 1998 providers at CARE felt that managed care had the potential to integrate delivery systems, increase accountability, and widen access to underserved population, two years later the only benefits of managed care were felt to be cost-containment and increased accountability. Only one respondent felt that "services seem to be more streamlined and a little better coordinated," and another felt services had increased (both respondents were administrators). The majority of respondents did not feel that managed care provided any benefits, or they shared the more cynical criticism of managed care as focused on managing money, not care.

Providers at CARE were quite outspoken in their identification of the problems with managed care. Most prevalent were their concerns over the quality of the care provided, and the limitations placed upon long-term services. Providers reported that patients were often discharged without adequate treatment, or they did not get the services needed. One nurse reported that managed care had resulted in:

shortened length of stay in the hospital for the seriously mentally ill, resulting in clients being ill and sent into the community before they are stabilized. The community resources are not in place for our client population, housing, and other supports . . . consequently clients get sick, they never stabilize, they have to return to the hospital—it's a revolving door.

The revolving door was associated with the early days of deinistitutionalization, when community supports for those with chronic and severe illnesses were nonexistent. However, now there are community supports, but providers cannot get authorization because treatment decisions are based primarily upon principles of cost-containment.

Table 5 contains the responses to the fixed-choice questions administered in 2000 about the effects of managed care on services. While some providers felt managed care affords an opportunity to develop a better system of mental health services (17.8 percent), a larger proportion disagreed with this statement (35.5 percent). Close to 80 percent disagreed that managed care had improved the quality of care; 64.4 percent disagreed that clinical outcomes had improved, and slightly over 50 percent felt that man-

Table 5. Attitudes Toward Managed Care (N=45, percentages)

	Disagree %	Neither %	Agree %
Managed care affords an opportunity to develop a better system of MH services.	35.5	24.4	17.8
With managed care, the quality of care available to clients has improved	77.8	11.1	11.1
With managed care, clinical outcomes for most clients has improved	64.4	24.4	11.1
Managed care inevitably results in underservice to clients	2.2	26.7	51.1

How often do financial considerations imposed by the various mechanisms to manage care result in the following for clients?

	Often	Sometimes	Never
Reduced use of community-based services	31.8	61.4	6.8
Reduced duration of treatment	52.3	40.9	6.8
Provide for a less intensive treatment than you would prefer	47.6	40.5	11.9
Greater reliance on medication than you would prefer	31.8	47.7	20.5
Reduced length of stay	56.8	38.6	4.5

aged care inevitably results in underservice to clients. Providers believed that the institutional logic of cost-containment (operationalized as the use of financial considerations to manage care) has resulted in reduced use of community-based services, reduced duration of treatment, less intensive treatment, a greater reliance on psychiatric medication than providers would prefer, and reduced length of outpatient care for clients.

A comparison of the service orientation between 1998 and 2000 supports the providers' perceptions that managed care is having a negative effect on the services available to their clients (Table 6). On every dimension of the Community Program Philosophy Scale, there was less emphasis on the provision of community-based care in 2000. An orientation toward community outreach, housing assistance, referral advocacy, and emergency access were all significantly lower in 2000, and there was significantly less emphasis on psychotherapy (or one-to-one counseling). Community outreach, housing assistance, referrals, and emergency access are all critical components of community-based care.

In describing how their work had changed since the advent of managed

Table 6. Changes in Community Program Philosophy*

	1998 N=51	2000 N=47
Outreach Orientation[c]	15.08 (2.46)	13.21 (2.42)
Team Model	14.71 (2.73)	14.17 (2.44)
Housing Assistance[a]	16.67 (1.77)	15.70 (3.04)
Interest in SMI Clients	15.04 (1.88)	14.72 (2.36)
Family Orientation	13.94 (3.26)	13.87 (2.66)
Substance Abuse Orientation	17.27 (1.48)	17.64 (6.75)
Linking to Entitlements	16.55 (2.10)	15.89 (2.83)
Referral Advocacy[a]	15.59 (2.23)	14.38 (2.78)
Interagency Orientation	14.63 (2.48)	14.30 (2.58)
Client Empowerment	15.43 (2.55)	14.57 (2.79)
Vocational Emphasis	15.29 (2.58)	14.91 (2.44)
Deemphasis on Psychotherapy[b]	12.90 (2.91)	14.70 (2.69)
Emphasis on Medication	17.69 (1.77)	17.55 (1.87)
Longitudinality of Service	16.16 (2.51)	16.08 (3.02)
Emergency Access[b]	13.74 (2.28)	12.25 (3.02)

*(scales range from 4 to 20, with higher score indicating agreement that the organization emphasizes this type of service or orientation).
[a]$p < .05$, [b]$p < .01$, [c]$p < .001$

care, providers at CARE universally complained about excessive paperwork and difficulties with the management information system. A nurse provider stated that,

> The paperwork has expanded at least four-fold, and is taking additional time from patient care. There is no time to build a relationship with a patient or his family, and trust is lost, the frustration level in providing care because of cumbersome preapproval procedures and denials of needed services has increase to a level where I will be glad to leave nursing.

Two case managers reported they "treat the computer, not the consumer," and the "human connection feels more automated; it's assembly line maintenance." Everyone reported spending less time with clients, and far more time meeting bureaucratic demands. Once again, these impressions are supported by the quantitative assessment of the work environment and work experiences (Table 7). Providers found the work environment to be less supportive of their work because of less job involvement, reduced role clarity, and lower levels of group cohesion. Providers also reported significantly less satisfaction with the nature of their work and less autonomy. While not statistically significant, providers experienced less input into de-

Table 7. Changes in Work Environment and Working Experiences
        Means and s.d

	1998 N=51	2000 N=47
Work Environment (all scales from 4 to 20; higher score indicates better work environment)		
Innovation	11.80 (3.46)	10.85 (3.80)
Involvement in Job[a]	14.35 (3.05)	12.91 (3.51)
Role Clarity[a]	13.24 (4.05)	11.15 (4.24)
Supervisory Support	13.57 (3.48)	12.49 (3.79)
Group Cohesion[a]	14.22 (2.99)	12.64 (3.89)
Work Experiences (higher score indicates better work experiences)		
Autonomy (2–5)[a]	3.56 (.68)	3.30 (.70)
Decision Input (0–9)	7.25 (2.67)	6.23 (2.45)
Job Involvement (2–4)	2.82 (.56)	2.70 (.53)
Satisfaction with Nature of Work (2–5)[b]	3.99 (.56)	3.65 (.75)
Satisfaction with Pay (1–4)	2.78 (.85)	2.67 (.78)
Satisfaction with Professional Status (2–5)	3.74 (.53)	3.60 (.56)
Satisfaction with Operating Procedures (1–5)	2.87 (.83)	2.65 (.77)
Burnout (higher score indicates higher levels of burnout)		
Emotional Exhaustion (0–6)[a]	1.86 (1.21)	2.42 (1.48)
Depersonalization (0–6)	1.01 (.98)	.92 (1.02)
Lack of Personal Accomplishment	1.00 (.72)	1.08 (.76)

[a]$p < .05$, [b]$p < .01$, [c]$p < .001$

cisions, lower levels of job involvement, and reduced satisfaction with pay, professional status, and operating procedures. Finally, providers also experienced higher levels of emotional exhaustion, or burnout.

It was also evident that providers at CARE felt a great deal of disillusionment; several responded to my question about how they thought their work would change in the next ten years with plans to leave mental health care: "I'm going to retire and escape this mess."

CONCLUSION

In this chapter I have examined the bureaucratic context of public sector mental health work. Providers value collaboration and a sense of teamwork, as well as the autonomy and freedom to make decisions about the

care needed by their clients. Managed care is indeed leading to a deprofessionalization of provider roles, and is increasing the power of the bureaucracy to make decisions about care. In addition to increasing the
amount of paperwork and decreasing the autonomy of providers, managed care may also exacerbate occupational and professional conflicts.
More fundamentally, managed care prevents providers from performing
the type of care they feel their clients need, and has led to a decrease in the
provision of the basic components of community-based care. This chapter
showed that providers had increased levels of burnout with managed care.
In the next chapter I examine the sources of burnout in mental health work.

NOTES

1. The term "behavioral healthcare" is often used to refer to mental health and
substance abuse services. Since the focus of this book is on mental health care, I use
that term rather than behavioral health.

2. However, Cook and Wright (1995) argue that the lack of an unambiguous
treatment technology actually gives mental health care professionals greater job
latitude.

3. Individual characteristics are also important (age, gender, etc.). For example,
Schaubroeck and Merritt (1997) found that in a test of Karasek's decision-control
model that feelings of self-efficacy affected perceptions of control and demands.

6 Exhausted Providers

Emotional Labor and Burnout

It's not the organization, but the emotional load of clients that causes burnout. The rest is ordinary stress—we all face that. Burnout is emotional load—overwhelmed with pain and hostility; people who carry a lot of pain—it adds to that emotional load. I see about 20 clients a week—that's all I can handle emotionally. (Private Clinician)

The last chapter showed that providers at CARE had higher levels of psychological burnout with the advent of managed care. In this chapter I focus on the providers' experience of psychological burnout. Psychological burnout (hereafter referred to as burnout) has been differentiated from job stress and job dissatisfaction to refer specifically to physical and emotional depletion caused by conditions of work in human service organizations, which can result in emotional detachment, cynicism, and deteriorating work performance (Cherniss 1980; Farber 1983; Jackson et al. 1986; Starrin et al. 1990). The central question behind much of the research on burnout is whether it is caused by the stress of caring for clients, or by the organization in which providers work. While Burke and Greenglass (1995, 1999) found that both individual characteristics and work stress predict burnout, most evidence points to the critical role played by the organization (Handy 1988; Meyerson 1994; Schulz et al. 1995). Scott et al. (1995: 84) argue that an unresponsive bureaucracy is "significantly more predictive of burnout than . . . emotional stressors inherent in the work itself." Consequently, burnout has been considered as a form of alienation—a reaction to the fragmentation of work and loss of autonomy engendered by bureaucratic work conditions (Farber 1983; McNeely 1983).

In this chapter I extend the understanding of burnout to include a consideration of emotional labor. Emotional labor occurs when "the emotional style of offering the service is part of the service itself" (Hochschild 1983: 5). Studies of emotional labor focus on the relational as opposed to the task aspects of a job (Steinberg and Figard 1999). Researchers studying emotional labor have analyzed the various ways in which organizations control the emotional labor of their employees in order to meet various organizational goals and have emphasized the relative lack of autonomy of the emotional laborer (Aches 1991; Aiken and Sloan 1997; Cherniss 1980; Handy 1988; Meyerson 1994). Typically, organizations require their emotional laborers to display emotions (i.e., friendliness, helpfulness) they do not necessarily feel (Hochschild 1983; Leidner 1993).

Mental health care workers must do more than maintain a smile or a friendly demeanor, they must also develop an intense, personal relationship that directly involves the emotions of their clients. In so doing, mental health care providers are subject to "strong, normative constraints" (Thoits 1990: 187). The emotional labor of providers involves caring work. Himmelweit (1999) argues that "caring" work is to be distinguished from other jobs involving emotional labor (for example, the flight attendants studied by Hochschild) by the fact that the emotional labor is not a cost but a desirable aspect of the job. With caring work providers manage their own feelings in order to obtain a desired state in another. Because of their professional training, those who perform caring labor *hold themselves* to normative standards that dictate a certain kind and degree of emotional labor (i.e., those feeling rules that are defined by a given treatment ideology).

The management, or organizational control, of emotional labor also causes burnout (Steinberg and Figard 1999). As mentioned above, feelings of inauthenticity and burnout result when the organization in which one works requires the worker to experience or express feelings they do not necessarily feel, or to control the expression of authentic feelings in order to achieve organizational goals. Most of the research on emotional labor has focused on various types of service workers who interact with customers. Fewer studies have focused on those in the caring profession (but see O'Brien 1994); consequently, England and Folbre (1999) call for more research on the relationship between caring labor and burnout. This chapter will show that what is unique about caring labor is the fact that the organization does not seek to control the emotional labor of its employees, but the organization in fact *prevents* the provider from performing the kinds of emotional labor the provider feels is needed by the client.

Standards governing emotional labor are professionally (or occupationally) dictated; that is, treatment ideologies specify the appropriate feeling rules or emotional norms that providers are expected to exhibit to their clients. As we have seen, treatment occurs within concrete organizational settings. Therefore, organizational working conditions can hinder or assist one's ability to perform emotional labor. Rather than controlling the emotional labor of providers, organizational conditions make it difficult for the provider to have the feelings and act in the way they have been trained to do. Hence, part of the experience of burnout for providers involves the traditional conflict between professional standards and bureaucratic constraints. I will first review the literature on burnout, and then provide a more thorough discussion of emotional labor, emphasizing the importance of emotional labor to the experience of burnout. Qualitative data from the providers at CARE, SUPPORT, and those in private practice are used to explore the meaning of burnout, and the centrality of emotional labor to provider's work.

BURNOUT IN MENTAL HEALTH WORK

Maslach (1982) provides the most concise overview of burnout and developed the Maslach Burnout Inventory (MBI). The MBI is the standard instrument for the empirical analysis of burnout and has even been used in global research (Golembiewski et al. 1996). Burnout is conceptualized in terms of three distinct dimensions: emotional exhaustion (an inability to feel compassion for clients), depersonalization (callousness toward clients), and a lack of personal accomplishment (a tendency to evaluate oneself negatively). Leiter (1991) states that emotional exhaustion is the *defining* feature of burnout, and if depersonalization and/or lack of personal accomplishment exist without emotional exhaustion, some process other than burnout is at play.[1]

Karasek and Theorell (1990) and Farber (1983) regard the symptoms of burnout as similar to those of depression or exhaustion, since burnout arises from the inability to meet socioemotional demands from one's clients or when these demands are excessive (Karasek and Theorell 1990). These definitions of burnout all point to the salience of emotional labor; emotional exhaustion and depersonalization both represent violations of the appropriate feeling rules because human service workers are expected to feel concern and compassion for their clients. A lack of personal accomplishment contributes to the most debilitating effect of burnout in which one's sense of self is negatively affected.

Williams (1989), in a study to determine if empathy and burnout were "polar" concepts, found that empathy was correlated with emotional exhaustion and depersonalization. Empathy is an obvious type of emotional labor that can be draining, producing the typical manifestations of burnout. Human service workers' involvement with needy people contributes to burnout and can result in a negative view of clients, a focus on the problems of clients, a lack of positive feedback, emotional stress, and overinvolvement with the clients' problems. The job setting contributes to burnout when work is distasteful or upsetting, caseloads are too high, or workers experience a lack of autonomy or difficult relations with coworkers and/or supervisors (Maslach 1982), all of which prevent the worker from meeting the demands stipulated by the emotional labor of clinical work. Hence, organizational structure is not itself the primary source of burnout, rather it is the *nature* of client demands that is a key factor in producing burnout (Cordes and Dougherty 1993: 642). As articulated by Burfoot (1994), the organization prevents the caregiver from attending to the needs of the client, who is thus not perceived by the caregiver to be a significant source of burnout; instead, the organization is targeted. Yet in fact, what distinguishes burnout from stress (which is produced by poor organizational working conditions) is that these stressors prevent the caregiver from attending to the needs of their clients. Hence, burnout is felt to arise from unmediated stress. But it is not simply stress; burnout occurs because the providers are not allowed to perform the needed emotional labor. Hence their professional identity, which is brought forth when engaged in emotional labor, is not fully realized in their work. It is not control over work, but the ability to *be* a certain kind of provider that is crucial to burnout. Thus burnout involves a unique type of autonomy.

Burnout affects the ability of the organization to perform (Price 1989) and is a significant predictor of turnover (Lake 1988); consequently, there has been a great deal of research on the conditions that cause burnout. Aiken and Sloan (1997) note that over one hundred factors have been found to be associated with burnout. "Bluntly, *anything* can be a precursor of burnout for *somebody* at *sometime*" (Golembiewski et al. 1996). Recent empirical assessments of burnout, both quantitative (Schulz et al. 1995) and qualitative (Meyerson 1994), attest to the critical role played by organizational context (see also Handy 1988). Role overload, role conflict, and role ambiguity are significant sources of stress in human service work and can lead to burnout (Cherniss 1980; Jayaratne and Chess 1983; Latack 1986; Motowidlo et al. 1986; Wolpin et al. 1991). Carney et al. (1993) found that case managers who were able to overcome organizational barriers and acquire resources for their clients, and who perceived support from the organization, experienced lower levels of burnout.

Mental health care providers experience higher levels of the factors that contribute to job stress and burnout (Cherniss 1980). There has been extensive research on burnout among mental health care workers (Kirk, et al. 1993; Reid et al. 1999; Sayers and Bond 2001; Schulz et al. 1995). As I showed in Chapter 2, the client population is especially demanding, yet there is a dearth of solutions or available programs to help providers meet the needs of their clients. There is also a notable lack of feedback from clients and little evidence of any concrete gains or improvement, especially among those with severe and persistent (or chronic) illnesses. In fact, these clients are often uncooperative and may not even acknowledge their problems, which can thwart efforts to provide care.

The structural sources of burnout may be heightened in the cases of providers who work with severely impaired clients. Role overload is a result of limited resources, client demands, and caseloads that are seen as too high. Role conflict occurs when caseworkers are expected to be all things for clients, or when the demands of the bureaucracy conflict with the providers' need to deal with each client individually. Role ambiguity is heightened by the lack of clearly defined treatment goals and positive feedback. Staff members are often left to their own devices to develop a guiding philosophy of treatment, yet the bureaucratic organization of many public service organizations may limit their power and autonomy (Cherniss 1980). In support of this line of reasoning, Finch and Krantz (1991) found relatively low levels of burnout and turnover among providers at Fountain House, an organization for the severely "mentally ill" with a clearly defined treatment philosophy and a participatory style of organizational management.

In summary, work with clients who have severe, persistent "mental illness" is likely to produce burnout, yet providers may derive great satisfaction from their work as long as the organizational structure does not prevent them from meeting the demands of their work role. However, the literature on burnout provides little theoretical articulation of what burnout *means* to providers, or how burnout is different from other types of organizational stress. I believe that burnout is best understood as a byproduct of emotional labor, which involves primarily norms and expectations about appropriate relationships with clients (i.e., treatment ideology). These norms specify the appropriate feeling rules associated with one's professional role and involve one's sense of self-identity. The critical variable is the providers' ability to meet the expectations of their professional identity, which is a broader type of autonomy than has been traditionally analyzed in studies of emotional labor and burnout.

EMOTIONAL LABOR AND IDENTITY

Emotional labor is associated with service work, namely, work that involves interactions with clients (as opposed to alienation that involves productive labor) and entails the management of feeling and the expression of appropriate emotions (Hochschild 1983). According to Hochschild (1989: 440) emotional labor is found when service workers "create and maintain a relationship, a mood, or a feeling." James (1989) also defines emotional labor as work that entails dealing with others' feelings in addition to regulating one's own feelings. The workers conform to feeling rules, which specify how they are to feel in a given situation.[2] The source of feeling rules are ideologies (Hochschild 1990), those systems of beliefs about how we are to act and behave. Treatment ideologies of providers are an important source of feeling rules.[3]

When workers manage their emotions, they engage in *surface acting*, a form of impression control in which they display emotions they do not necessarily feel, and *deep acting*, in which they actually feel the emotions expressed, which therefore calls for a greater investment of self. Because feelings are managed, emotional labor can affect our sense of identity. "This kind of labor calls for coordination of mind and feeling, and it sometimes draws on a source of self we honor as deep and integral to our individuality" (Hochschild 1983: 7).

Emotional demands can result in emotional exhaustion (Morris and Feldman 1996), but burnout involves more than the frequency of emotional display or the variety of emotions exhibited. Because emotions and feelings must be managed, emotional labor affects one's sense of identity and can precipitate unique conflicts between individuals and their occupational role identities. According to Hochschild (1983), emotion workers who identify wholeheartedly with their work roles risk burnout. Emotional labor calls for self-investment (Ashforth and Humphrey 1993) and thus is likely to produce burnout, which is a *unique* form of stress because one's identity is fundamentally compromised. Wharton (1993) also argues that burnout is a consequence of emotional labor (though her empirical analysis demonstrates that the relation between emotional labor and burnout is conditioned by a variety of other factors, including autonomy). Recent research has made the linkage between emotional labor and burnout explicit (Brotheridge and Grandy 2002; Erickson and Ritter 2001; Sapf et al. 2001; Scheid 1999a).

Ashforth and Humphrey (1993) extend Hochschild's original formulation to consider the various ways in which role identity moderates some of the negative effects of emotional labor. Specifically, those who strongly identify with their work roles are more likely to feel authentic when they are conforming to the demands of emotional labor. However, Ashforth and Humphrey (1993) concur with Hochschild (1983) that overidentification with one's role can lead to burnout. Other researchers who have examined the relationship between emotional labor and authenticity (Bulen et al. 1997; Erickson 1995) found that when organizations impose rules governing emotional display, workers are likely to feel inauthentic. Hence the crucial intervening process is the degree of autonomy workers have over their work roles.[4]

Van Maanen and Kunda also focus on the way organizational culture is used to produce the appropriate display of emotion; they hypothesize that when more emotional labor is required in a given work role, a higher investment of self is necessary, and work identity becomes more troublesome (1989: 54). Burnout is a consequence of the degree of emotional labor required to effectively perform the job and the degree to which one's conception of self is tied in to one's role identity. Van Maanen and Kunda (ibid.) also hypothesize that workers with greater job security, or who have higher pay and status, are more likely to support the feeling rules that go with the job. Consequently, older and more experienced workers and those who have advanced farther have been found to experience less burnout (Cordes and Dougherty 1993).

The importance of identity has been recognized by those who have examined the relationship between emotional labor and feelings of authenticity (Bulen et al. 1997; Erickson 1995; Erickson and Wharton 1997; Leidner 1993). Erickson and Ritter (2001) introduce the idea of the management of agitation as part of emotional labor, and find that higher levels of agitation contribute both feelings of inauthenticity and burnout. Bulen et al. (1997: 238) argue that the "identity dilemma may be aggravated further by employee's lack of control over the work role or becoming estranged from the interactional process itself." While important, this research has been limited by its focus on service workers who deal with the public.

Ashforth and Humphrey (1993) concur with the idea that some effects of emotional labor are moderated by the degree to which one identifies with one's work role. However, they emphasize only one aspect of emotional labor, surface acting, which is akin to Goffman's notion of impression management (i.e., we smile at customers even if they are rude). Hochschild (1983: 216) critiques Goffman for his focus on surface acting at the expense of the more important idea of deep acting: "Deep acting is not empirically alive in Goffman's work, and the theoretical statement about it is correspondingly weaker."

The analysis of emotional labor in terms of surface acting is a common theme in the research on emotional labor and its consequences; emphasis has been placed on those emotional laborers who are required by either their job or the organization to display emotions they do not necessarily feel (Bulen et al. 1997; Leidner 1993; Lively 2002; Pogrebin and Poole 1995; Saxton et al. 1991; Stenross and Kleinman 1989). Yet much emotional labor involves deep acting in which the worker must actually feel the emotions called forth by the job. Thus, professional role identity involves an investment of self. Organizations influence and shape the feelings of their members, profoundly affecting self-identity: "When work involves emotional commitment, individual members are likely to develop a self image organized around their occupational role" (Trice 1993: 37).

The emotional labor produced by providers is typical of deep acting; clinicians draw upon emotional memory and actually experience the emotion they are to display with clients (i.e., concern, regret, empathy). Providers (and other human service workers) are care givers and must be responsive emotionally (as well as intellectually and physically) to their clients. "Caregiving is a balancing act of attachment to, and detachment from others" (Kahn 1993: 554). This work demands that providers develop and maintain meaningful relationships. These relationships involve accessibility, inquiry, attention, validation, empathy, support, compassion, and consistency (Kahn 1993). Such deep acting fundamentally involves "self" and "identity" in a way that surface acting does not. Providers and other professional service workers learn emotional work via professional socialization (education, workshops, training programs, work experiences) which teaches them to deal effectively with clients (a process that involves emotional labor in itself) as well as to apply clinical techniques. Through professional socialization feeling rules are internalized, reducing the likelihood of conflict between the emotions dictated by "feeling rules" and one's "true feelings," thus curtailing emotional dissonance.

Rafaeli and Sutton (1989) argue that when feeling rules are internalized, workers still exhibit a degree of detachment, but their faking is in "good faith" and can enhance well-being. That is, professionals learn that some degree of detachment is necessary if they are to fulfill the emotional demands of their caring roles effectively. If providers become overinvolved with clients (a lack of detachment) or too detached (hardened and cynical) they risk psychological burnout and will be less competent caregivers as a result. Hence, professional norms specify the appropriate feelings rules (i.e., the emotions necessary to performance of a specific work role) as well as providing some guidance on how to avoid the negative consequences of emotional labor. I turn now to providers' accounts of their emotional labor, burnout, and the ways in which their organization helped them to prevent, or deal with, burnout.

EMOTIONAL LABORERS

I rely primarily upon the in-depth interviews with providers from CARE and SUPPORT, as well as interviews with private clinicians, to explore the meaning of burnout and emotional labor. It is important to note that when I first began interviewing providers, I did not have a preconceived view of burnout as a response to emotional labor; in fact, I did not view clinical work as typical of emotional labor. However, as I analyzed the data emotional labor emerged as a salient feature of mental health work. Consequently, in subsequent interviews, I probed more deeply into the nature of the providers' relationship with their work as well as their experience of burnout, both in their current work organization and in previous mental health care settings.[5]

Table 8 presents a summary of the typical symptoms of stress and burnout experienced by the providers who completed questionnaires. This is a standard set of descriptive questions (Cherniss 1980) and allows for some quantitative comparison of the experience of burnout. Providers at CARE and SUPPORT had similar symptoms of stress and burnout, as would be expected since they work with similar kinds of clients and perform similar kinds of emotional labor. Providers in private practice had

Table 8. Symptoms of Stress and Burnout
(Percentage Responding Yes)

Have you ever experienced any of the following in your current position?	PROVIDERS		
	CARE N=41	SUPPORT N=24	Private Practice N=22
Resistance to going to work every day	46.3	45.8	18.2
A sense of failure	34.1	45.8	9.1
Anger or resentment	61.0	62.2	45.5
Discouragement or indifference	56.1	54.2	45.5
Tired or exhausted all day	51.2	58.3	22.7
Loss of positive feelings toward clients	24.4	37.5	9.1
Postponing/resisting client contacts	26.8	29.2	22.7
Stereotyping clients	24.4	16.7	18.2
Inability to concentrate/listen to what client is saying	31.7	45.8	13.6
Cynicism toward clients/blaming them	22.0	20.8	9.1

much lower levels of stress and burnout, although they were as likely to engage in some types of distancing from their clients (i.e., postponing client contacts or stereotyping clients). It is notable that a significant proportion of all the providers interviewed had experienced anger or resentment and while the data does not explain why this is so, the qualitative data described below reveals that their anger is not directed at clients, but at various types of organizational constraints on the care provided.

One important aspect of emotional labor and burnout that has received much attention is the role played by gender. Service work often consists of traditionally female occupations (i.e., nurses) and much of the emotional labor is performed by women. Hochschild (1990) has increasingly come to analyze emotional labor in terms of gender strategies. While care giving work is typically seen as feminine, mental health care providers do more than provide care, and the role of therapist or case manager is not stereotypically "feminine" in the same way as the work of nurse is. Care giving is only one approach to mental health treatment; and Chapter 3 shows that female providers were more likely than male providers to describe their treatment role as that of care giver. However, male and female providers do not differ in their descriptions of burnout or emotional labor, and the relevant reports come equally from male and female providers. Furthermore, in quantitative analysis of burnout at CARE and SUPPORT (Andresky 1996) gender was not found to be significant.

I begin with the first time I heard providers discussing burnout.

Providers at CARE attended a series of retreats in the summer of 1992 (to which I was a nonparticipant observer), and one focus of the retreat was burnout. A large picture of the "Burned-Out Secretary" was placed in front of the group, and providers were asked to replace the descriptors for the "Burned-Out Secretary" with the "Burned-Out Clinician." Each department developed their own picture, which I then merged to create a composite sketch. The composite sketch of the "Burned-Out Clinician" developed during the retreats at CARE illustrated the workers' experience of burnout and provided a good start for a discussion of emotional labor and burnout. The themes described were expressed by many providers and engendered agreement or reflected common experiences.

The "Burned-Out Clinician" composite is an experientially based understanding of stress and burnout that is grounded in the context of providing for those with severe, persistent "mental illnesses" in a public mental health center. Providers experienced the emotional pressures of having to *smile* constantly and *listen* to clients, the urge to *punch* somebody, bad *nerves*, constant calls, ongoing crises, brown-nosing. These experiences illustrate the feeling rules required of the provider's role. At some times emotional labor is directed toward the client; at others it is directed toward other professionals with whom providers must interact. In sum, the provider is expected to be caring, to exhibit concern and empathy, solve all the problems faced by clients and to do so in a supportive manner.

Providers at CARE also described hair-raising experiences of violence and travel into "bad" neighborhoods. The constant interruptions of having clients and/or their families calling all day and the never-ending crises were salient features of a work environment that was described more than once as a "pressure cooker." Providers also expressed a degree of cynicism toward clients, claiming to be hard of hearing or having a "bleeding heart from clients' sob stories" or being pulled in too many directions by clients' needs: "I want," "I need," "Gimmee." The "Burned-Out Clinician" was given a bag stuffed with equipment that illustrated the providers' need to be ready for anything at any time (mace, Lysol®, bus tokens, cigarettes, condoms). Providers often attempted to gain some distance from emotional demands of their roles by exhibiting cynicism toward clients.

One story told at a retreat illustrates the cynicism that providers at one time or another experience:

> I took a call at 3 A.M. and the client said, "I'm trying to kill myself and I drank two gallons of paint." My first response was, "What color was the paint?" (Female MSW case manager)

Another provider added to this response, saying, "Two gallons wouldn't work, you need to drink two gallons more." The group laughed. This is not to suggest that providers are callous or uncaring, but rather that the constant demands of clients who need assistance with every facet of their lives, from grocery shopping and riding the bus to needing a therapist in times of crisis can produce the emotional exhaustion and depersonalization characteristic of burnout. Chambliss (1996) also describes the humor used by nurses to help them gain some distance from the often gruesome and painful reality of hospital work. Humor and cynicism are techniques that human service workers use to gain the necessary distance from their emotionally demanding work.

The majority of providers at both sites described their work role in terms of emotional labor, as having to maintain some kind of relationship with clients. This placed various types of emotional demands on the provider whereby they felt compelled to "be a total person involved with the full spectrum of another's needs," and had to work hard to "figure out the relationship" with each of their clients:

> I try to support people to live full lives and stay in the community, to be appreciated for their quirkiness, whatever . . . and that involves working with people on virtually every aspect of their lives. (Female nurse case manager)

Many providers identified active listening and feeling compassion for their clients as the key components of their work role. In response to the query, "What kinds of skills do you bring to your clinical role?" one respondent described the nature of the emotional relationship with his clients:

> One is an ability to listen . . . another is genuineness—I relate to people one-to-one, and so gaining their trust and confidence I work through relationships—why should somebody do something unless they have a motivation that involves a sense of I'll do this with you—for you—because I care about you. (Male MSW case manager)

Providers used descriptors of their work roles which clearly indicate that the work performed constitutes emotional labor. Providers were "caretakers" and "parents," "friends" and "advocates" (see Chapter 3 for a thorough discussion of these treatment roles). As such, providers sought to provide a haven in the community for their clients, to support their clients with a sense of belonging and security. Treatment involved "a lot of support, encouragement, listening, and trust-building," which can often lead to dependency and the fear that the provider may "do too much care taking." Other clinicians sought to empower their clients and help them develop needed survival skills that would lead to greater self-sufficiency. Providers also acted as advocates, going out on a limb to keep their clients out of the hospital (or prison), and fought to secure income, housing, and other forms of community support for their clients. All these roles require the development and maintenance of a relationship with the client, a relationship that draws upon one's self-identity and entails the management of feeling (that is, deep acting).

The critical incidents reported by providers at both sites also provide concrete examples of how mental health care is emotionally demanding. One-half of the providers described incidents that exemplified the positive role they played in a clients' recovery and generally reflected the client's achieving a degree of stability in the community after a long history of failure. These stories underscored the positive rewards of developing a good relationship with a client who had learned to experience trust. One provider (whose experience is typical) put a lot of effort into developing a "relationship with [a client], and developing trust, and I have felt very good about how well it's gone." Another provider said:

> He has trust in me and believes in me. It's been really emotional working with him, and to go through these ups and downs with him. (Male MSW case manager)

These providers described critical incidents that were not merely negative, but also reflected despair and pain over their involvement in the lives of their clients. This often occurred when "the bottom falls out, and you have to be there to pick up the pieces without being judgmental." Success stories, in which the client actually attains specified treatment goals, are the "exception in this type of work . . . there's not a lot of positive change . . . you are making baby steps all the time." Many stories told of violence and sometimes death: female clients' being raped or beaten, a client's child abused by a "normal" boyfriend. Another common theme was male clients who were violent, or had a gun and were "acting out" their aggression in situations that put the provider at some risk. Suicide threats and deaths due to suicide or violence was another sort of story that many providers "had a hard time shaking," or that created difficult emotional demands for the clinician.

"Typically" a provider's work entails a high degree of emotional involvement, and frequent incidents of emergency, violence, and death. Effective coping with this form of occupational stress calls for further emotional labor: remaining calm when faced with a threatening situation; maintaining composure at news of a client's death; avoiding being overly critical or judgmental about lifestyles and choices different from one's own; expressing care and concern for the misfortunes of one's clients; avoiding communicating a sense of helplessness and frustration to clients when the system lacks the resources to provide basic necessities. The costs of such labor can be emotional exhaustion, depersonalization, and lack of a sense of personal accomplishment.

The lack of personal accomplishment characteristic of burnout points to the role played by identity in understanding the unique sources of burnout. As Hochschild (1983) articulates, emotional labor involves one's sense of self, one's identity. For providers, work role and identity are closely connected. Almost all of the providers I interviewed closely identified with their work, with their clients, and with the wider social good of helping others.

> I'm a person who needs to make an investment. My work isn't just a paycheck, my work is everything to me, and I need to feel like I'm making a difference. (Female MSW case manager)

> Part of my self-concept is bolstered because I work with people who have serious mental illness, they are folks in real need. . . . This kind of work feeds my needs to feel like I am doing important work. (Female nurse provider)

When providers felt burned out, they no longer had that kind of positive identification with their work, and experienced the loss of personal accomplishment where they were "just looking forward to the end of the day."

> There is this sense of a big looming dark abyss, and I'm going to walk into it every day. There may be some silver linings, but there is this backdrop of dark clouds. (Male case manager)

The data showed burnout to be an inability to give the needed emotional labor. It was a consequence of giving too much emotional support: "I just couldn't take anymore in; I just didn't care." Providers who described themselves as having burnout felt an overwhelming sense of responsibility for their clients: "I would begin to feel very overwhelmed, scared and guilty." Or: "Case managers are very involved with their clients, they have a difficult time saying no, and that can become overwhelming." One provider felt burnout was a direct consequence of the therapist's "taking on more responsibility for the work of therapy than the client." According to another provider,

> Burnout is an attitude, negative, disrespectful. No tolerance for clients, no ability to be objective. I worry about burnout because I'm a pretty emotional person. I do think you have to keep that wall up. Me, I get connected to clients, I emotionally connect. (Female MSW case manager)

Providers in private practice also experienced burnout.

> For me, depression sets in. I feel a lack of energy, a type of drain. There are days when I leave the office after some horrendous account of abuse, or something God awful that happened because of someone's addiction, and it's so draining. Its hard to hear that day after day. (Female PhD psychologist)

Keeping the wall up, learning to "make a distinction and let go, to not take it to bed," means developing some distance between the emotional demands made by clients and one's sense of self and identity. Providers knew they had to develop coping mechanisms, to not let their work overwhelm them. One external condition that could assist, or hinder, the clinicians with meeting the emotional demands of their work role was the organization in which they worked.

ORGANIZATIONAL CONSTRAINTS
ON EMOTIONAL LABOR

The written responses to the request, "Please write a brief description of when you feel stressed in your job," reveal both the organizational and occupational aspects of stress. Supervisors felt stressed at the end of the month when a variety of reports were due or when staff did not follow procedures, or they worry over the lack of resources. Nurses reported stress due to overbooking of medication appointments or conflicts with doctors and case managers. Case managers mentioned paperwork; every time they see a client a report has to be filed. Organizational requirements often conflicted with the provider's primary role:

> I feel stressed when I can't do all the paperwork required unless I don't see my clients as necessary. If I see my clients as frequently as required I can't do the paperwork. (Female case manager)

The majority of the providers at both CARE and SUPPORT targeted multiple demands and the persistent feeling of being behind in one's work as primary sources of stress. "When there are too many things to do and not enough time," and when "they all feel like priorities." This is typical of stress in most work settings where the demands of the job are overwhelming.

Compounding the problem of multiple demands, caseloads were universally felt to be too high: 30 to 35 per case manager at CARE and primary responsibility for 12 to 15 and team support for another 20 or so at SUPPORT. With this many clients, daily crises (suicide threats, emergency hospitalization, arrests, housing, referrals, job placements) are organizational facts of life and lead to a work environment that is characterized as a pressure cooker.

> I feel stressed *every day* as clients are in the building 7–8 hours all day long. Most of them are so needy. They are constantly *with* you—even follow us to the bathroom demanding attention. Even office space is not private as clients are constantly "in and out" seeing, talking, or asking something of one of us.

We "live" with the population everyday. We need more space, more hours in the day, more energy to respond to the demands. (Female case manager)

Providers in private practice targeted control over one's caseload as central to the management of emotional labor. Twenty clients a week appeared to be the magic number; but also important was the *type* of client seen. As noted, providers in public MHOs work primarily with clients with severe, persistent mental illnesses. Several of the providers in private practice that I interviewed had left public mental health care for private practice because of this exclusive work with severe illnesses:

I had a lot of difficulty with our public system's moving toward having only specialty populations for our clinicians. I didn't want 100 percent of my clients to be one type of diagnosis—it's the variety that keeps you from burning out. (Male MSW therapist)

Private clinicians were in a position to limit their caseloads (while they did experience a loss of income, most felt they did very well), and they could also select the type of client they would work with. "I'm very choosy about my clients," was a common refrain.

Providers in the public MHOs did not have much ability (or power) to select their clients, and therefore experienced a degree of frustration with some of them. One provider summarized the general feeling of frustration about clients as follows: "When I work hard, make contacts, go out on a limb, and break my neck setting up something for the client's benefit and the client doesn't follow through." Yet most providers did not blame their clients for burnout; rather, they felt that such difficulties in providing care and support were what the job naturally entailed:

Consumers rarely cause me to be stressed. Working with and for them makes this job worthwhile. The politics of the organization is a major stress. Personally I have minimal empowerment and I feel this is true for most people in my position. (Female MSW case manager)

The following description exemplifies how the provider is overwhelmed by both multiple demands and too many clients, and also demonstrates how stress can be amplified or diminished by the organizational conditions of work:

I feel stressed when so much is required of me by so many different people at the same time. I work with the client, the family, the community, the mental health system, etc. It's sometimes very draining to be the sounding board for all these people. I especially become resentful when clients, their families, doctors sometimes forget how many clients are on my caseload and how many hours are in one day! My supervisor is very supportive and keeps me going because of this. (Female case manager)

It is not just work with clients or role overload, but also the emotional demands involved in providing care to clients that produces the emotional exhaustion (expressed by this clinician as feeling "drained") characteristic of burnout. Another provider stated that burnout is a result of the organization not providing the worker with the necessary resources and support to meet the emotional demands of their role:

> I got burned out from the system because the system [a previous job] wasn't doing anything to protect me . . . that burned me out—a helplessness—a powerlessness—feeling like somebody is putting a leash on you. (Male MSW case manager)

In their analysis of intensive case managers, Carney et al. (1993) found that the ability to overcome organizational barriers and acquire resources for clients reduced burnout. The organization can also help shield the worker from the negative effects of emotional labor (Stenross and Kleinman 1989). These generalizations received strong support from the responses of the providers at SUPPORT, who had been asked to differentiate stress from burnout and to identify the sources of burnout as well as the factors that helped alleviate burnout.

Burnout was described as a feeling of isolation, and providers blamed their supervisor or colleagues for failing to provide them with the organizational supports they needed to deal with the demands of emotional labor.

> A lack of support from supervisors contributes to my feeling burnout and leads to a feeling of helplessness, hopelessness. Feeling isolated from the team as though I don't have team assistance with a difficult client leads to burnout. Things that help alleviate burnout are teamwork, sharing responsibility for difficult clients, and a team that functions in healthy ways. (Female MSW case manager)

Burnout was differentiated from stress in that burned-out workers no longer felt able to do the job well, or were prevented from doing their job due to oppressive work conditions or a bureaucratic supervisor. Burnout was described as "feeling tapped on energy," "not giving a damn anymore," "no creative ideas," or "not being listened to, not being respected."

> Burnout is an overall giving up, and losing the commitment and focus on the type of work, and the people we work with. It is so draining—this type of work. Programmatic and management factors play a big role. (Female case manager)

> It's a feeling of not giving a damn anymore, if someone walks in and sits next to me, it's not my problem. I think the genesis of it is stress—expectations

that are unrealistic that by and large part are placed on staff by program managers. Working with clients can be very stressful—but that has to be given top priority, it has to be given support. There has to be a level of understanding that the clinical work comes first—dealing with the person, not the paperwork. (Male case manager)

Hochschild (1983) argues that meeting the demands of emotional labor are intensified when the worker lacks control over the conditions of work. According to Cherniss (1980) psychological success (feeling of predictability and control) is hindered by the bureaucratic conditions of many organizations, and contributes to the experience of burnout. Similarly, providers found organizational conditions exacerbated the difficulties generated by the emotional labor required to successfully provide care to clients. They specifically identified ineffective organizational supports, especially on the part of supervisors, as the primary source of burnout. For providers, the principal source of burnout is not the attempts of the organization to control their emotional labor, but rather, the ability of the organization to prevent them from performing the necessary emotional labor to care for clients.

A feeling I am not accomplishing anything worthwhile especially when someone is preventing me from pursuing things my own way. (Female MSW case manager)

I am certain this was not caused by the clients, but rather by very inadequate support from my supervisor. I did not have enough control about treatment decisions with my clients. (Female case manager)

As providers are all caregivers, that is, emotional laborers, they are not likely to target emotional labor as the primary source of their burnout. Instead, as also found by Burfoot (1994) in her study of nurses, providers identified organizational variables as critical, because the organization prevented them from fulfilling the demands of their work roles. Furthermore, the factors that alleviated burnout identified by providers in the public realm were all organizational: a good supervisor, team support, frequent vacations, and good pay, which contributed to a sense that one's efforts were validated. As articulated by one provider, "if you are getting support from your supervisor, or the team, then the client issues don't bother you nearly so much." Providers in private practice avoided burnout by limiting the number of clients, or restricting the type of clients they saw.

One provider I interviewed had indeed burned-out in her private practice. She left mental health after twenty years because

I didn't have the type of clients whom I felt good about after they left. I didn't have easy clients anymore. I noticed I was getting tearful, having a lot more problems separating from the stuff people were telling me, and it just seemed like it was time.

CONCLUSION

I have argued that emotional labor is critical to the experience of burnout, but not predictive of it. Rather, burnout should be thought of as the failure of emotional labor. It is likely to result when organizations either seek to control the conditions under which emotional labor is performed, the emotional labor itself, or when the organization does not adequately support the emotional labor of their employees. The organization can assist the workers with their emotional labor by providing support (either from coworkers or supervisors), or by providing opportunities that enable them to maintain some distance from their work role (such as a team model or adequate vacation time).

Burnout can also result from the organization's attempts to control the ways in which an individual acts and feels (both surface and deep acting). For example, some mental health organizations advocate a type of reality therapy in which the clinician is expected to act as a stern parent: rewarding positive behavior and punishing negative behavior in various ways. A provider whose professional and/or personal identity is one of "friend" or "advocate" would not be able to meet the feeling rules dictated by the organization and would be likely to experience burnout. Similarly, the speed-up (multiple demands or simply too many clients) creates an organizational context likely to produce a sense of stress, because the emotional laborer is prevented from meeting professionally prescribed feeling rules, resulting in burnout. The next chapter examines how the commodification of care under managed care has affected providers' sense of control over their work, and, consequently, their levels of burnout.

NOTES

1. Wallace and Brinkerhoff (1991) have raised questions about the theoretical and empirical validity of the depersonalization and lack of personal accomplishment indices. Many processes other than burnout may be at work when providers report a sense of depersonalization or a lack of personal accomplishment.

2. Hochschild (1990) differentiates between display rules, which govern how we are to appear in a given social interaction, and feeling rules, which govern how we are to feel.

3. Soderfeldt et al. (1996: 1224) also targets "ideological definitions of responsibilities and arenas for action" as important to understanding strain in human service work. As I argued in the introduction, treatment ideologies (and the match

between individual- and organizational-level beliefs) are important to understanding both job satisfaction and burnout.

4. As noted in the previous chapter, Schaubroeck and Merritt (1997) found self-efficacy to be central to perceptions of control; self-efficacy is certainly critical to understanding one's identity and feelings about how one meets the demands of emotional labor.

5. This is especially critical for private clinicians, the majority of whom had prior work experiences in public agencies, and often left the public realm for private practice precisely because they were "burned out."

7   The Commodification of Care

Getting on the phone and asking for sessions, having to do assessments, having to write up all kinds of information . . . they are just putting another layer
of bureaucracy in there and they are having to pay more people to be on the
other end of the phones (MSW private therapist)

In managed care, with its emphasis upon cost-containment, performance-
assessment, and measurable mental health outcomes, the treatment actions of providers are subject to increased scrutiny and organizational
control. What happens when treatment decisions are made by third-party
payers whose principal motivation is cost savings? What happens when
providers are not allowed to give the type of care they have learned is
professionally appropriate and necessary to achieve the mental health
outcomes their clients seek? More fundamentally, how do providers experience the conflict between their professional logics of care and the commodification of care?

Smith (1992) studied the emotional labor of nursing at the beginning of
the Thatcher reforms to the British National Health Service. In a recent essay (1999) she speculates about whether the privatization of health care
will result in the commercialization of emotional labor, and details the importance of supportive organizational arrangements that enable nurses to
perform their emotional labor. In a recent study of the effect of managed
care on hospital physicians, Hoff et al. (2002) find that the quality of relationships with colleagues and patients has more effect on burnout than the
type of fiscal and clinical restraints imposed by managed care. Of course,
doctors do tend to maintain a high degree of control over clinical decisions
by virtue of their professional expertise (Griffiths and Hughs 1999; Hoff
and McCaffrey 1996; Weiss and Fitzpatrick 1997).

The critical factor that affects the providers' ability to do their work in
accordance with their own professional logics of care is the degree of autonomy and control they have over treatment decisions. Autonomy allows

the provider to perform necessary emotional labor in the manner to which they have been socialized to believe is appropriate. Yet managed care represents a direct threat to the autonomy of mental health care providers. First I look at the experience of the private clinicians whom I interviewed and who completed questionnaires, because their work has been subject to more overt mechanisms to manage care than has the work of providers in the public sector. Then I examine how managed care has changed the work experiences of providers at CARE.

EXTERNAL CONTROL OF THERAPEUTIC CARE

Managed care has had a radical effect on the work of private therapists; many of the providers interviewed seriously consider leaving private practice if they cannot find ways to circumvent the restrictions imposed by managed care entities and third-party insurers. On average, about 50–80 percent of the clients seen by providers in private practice were covered by some form of managed care. Providers reported they deal with an average of four to five different managed care companies. As shown in Chapter 4, managed care has changed both the types of clients seen by providers as well as the types of services they provide.

While some therapists acknowledge that managed care has the potential to improve both access to care and the effectiveness of that care, the prevailing sentiment is that managed care imposes a significant barrier to quality care. As one family therapist described managed care: "It is a proven way to slow the therapeutic process down until clients get so disgruntled they leave therapy, often prematurely." This same therapist went on to articulate the central conflict posed by managed care:

> Managed care breaches the confidentiality of the therapeutic process and alters the relationship between the patient and the therapist. Insurance companies have totally different goals, like bottom line profitability, than what the therapist and client have in their contract for change.

The conflict was a significant source of stress. When asked on the written questionnaire distributed in 1998 to identify when they felt *most stressed* in their work, 36.4 percent of the clinicians in private practice identified client-related problems, 27.3 percent targeted managed care hassles, and another 14 percent cited paperwork. Managed care has created "more hoops for the client to jump through and for me the therapist to jump through as well" (Female MSW therapist). The major source of frustration was when managed care companies denied what providers felt was necessary treatment. An MSW therapist felt stressed when managed care will not give a client hospitalizations or sessions when they need it, and they make it hard to start up groups, there is too much paperwork and time on the phone. They waste time, create barriers to treatment, and end treatment too early.

Managed care has increased the amount of paperwork and time spent on the phone getting authorization for treatment or additional sessions. As such it has effectively added another layer of bureaucracy, and the majority of the providers identified negotiating with managed care companies and completing unnecessary paperwork as those aspects of their job they most disliked. The documentation required by managed care was felt to be "excessive" and it took time away not only from client care, but also from the continuing education of the therapist. Not only was the amount of paperwork "time-consuming, redundant, and unhelpful to the therapeutic process," the information requested by many managed care companies "compromised confidentiality" (Female psychological associate).

The overwhelming issue with managed care concerned the threats to client confidentiality and quality care. Utilization and oversight review were felt to constitute a clear assault on client confidentiality, and providers in private practice recognized the significant challenge to their own professional expertise and autonomy as well as the freedom of their clients to select their own therapist. Patient privacy rights were also violated by third-party requests for detailed information in order to justify treatment. More ominous were the denials of care; providers found managed care produces situations in which "people are denied needed care all the time" (MSW therapist).

Far more common than an outright denial of care were restrictions placed on the number of sessions, and the providers' knowledge that if they asked too often for more sessions they would be dropped from that insurer's panel. Providers described the limitations imposed on authorized sessions as "premature termination" because the clients were often unable to afford to continue treatment on their own. While therapists were generally willing to continue treatment at reduced fees, such practices were explicitly outlawed by their contract with the managed care company. Providers resented the process of utilization review, and were frustrated by having to deal with those companies that "dole out one to three sessions at a time" (PhD psychoanalyst). They also raised questions about the qualifications of managed care case managers, many of whom appeared to be only "insurance clerks" to whom a provider had to disclose personal and often confidential information in order to obtain authorization for therapy. "Negotiating for sessions with managed care" was felt to be noxious "because it's not about care." Rather, managed care had "control of access to mental health care" in the name of corporate profits (Female PhD psychoanalyst).

In addition to limiting care to clients, managed care had changed the types of services therapists could provide to their clients, as shown in Chapter 4. One female MSW therapist summarizes:

> People doing in-depth work [with clients] have had to quit due to limited visits and lower payments. Managed care clients tend to be more crises-oriented and less psychologically sophisticated. I do more crisis counseling, more cognitive-behavioral counseling rather than analytically-oriented, object-relating, insight therapy. Managed care is more focused and goal-oriented. The major problem here is that the goal seems to be profit for the CEO at the expense of providers and patients.

There was also less emphasis on evaluation, or testing, "as this is never approved" by managed care companies. While some clinicians liked having some short-term clients in their caseload, they were concerned about those clients that need long-term therapy, and their inability to get such care approved by a managed care insurer. These restrictions on care had led one provider to feel "anger and resentment over the injustice of a broker who is making money off my labor and is draining my life-blood and energy." This provider is clearly burned out.

One-half of the private practice clinicians who completed the questionnaire said that they had experienced burnout, and over 70 percent of these targeted managed care as the source of their burnout. Burnout was due to "having to cope with the other client—the insurance company, it has produced a sense of helplessness and a lack of control over my work" (Male PhD psychologist).

> Burnout is due to toxic environments—those with too much emphasis on productivity and numbers, little individual consideration of cases, increasing pressures for uniformity (Female psychologist)

Not surprisingly, providers sought ways to circumvent the restrictions of managed care and to create ways to stay in private practice. About one-fourth of those who had been interviewed and who had completed the questionnaire no longer worked with managed care. In their response to the query, "How do you prevent burnout?" several providers were quite blunt: "I need to stop doing managed care." Several well-established providers were able to avoid managed care companies and maintain a traditional fee-for-service practice, though they acknowledged their clients were wealthier and had different needs. "I no longer work with managed care; consequently my caseload tends to be upper middle class" (Female MSW therapist). Some providers had a unique "niche" or area of specialization (e.g., substance abuse, sexual dysfunction, or couples therapy), which allowed them to continue their traditional way of providing services. Others tried to maintain some sense of professional and personal integrity. One PhD psychologist stated that burnout could only be prevented by his ability to maintain

> A broad perspective of my work as my life work; this involves a spiritual perspective where work is placed in the broader context of meaningful life activity. The value of my work is defined internally, not by some insurance payment rate.

Of particular interest was evidence of organized resistance to managed care. A number of providers had formed group practices with the stated mission that they did not deal with managed care. One such group, identified themselves as a professional consortium whose mission statement reads as follows:

> The mission of __ is to uphold the integrity of the psychotherapy process in the changing mental health care market place through informed treatment, privacy, and freedom of choice. Members are committed to the concept that treatment should meet the needs primarily of the client rather than the health care system. Treatment should be short-term and symptom-focused when it is appropriate to patient need and desire. Likewise, when appropriate to patient need and desire, treatment should continue long enough to meet the client's needs and to reach his/her goals.

In addition to psychotherapy, the consortium also provided referral services and worked with clients to select the right therapist and helped educate them about therapy, "including how it may be shaped and impacted by intervening third parties of many types." Such efforts are evidence of countervailing power, and constitute a direct challenge to the authority of managed care companies.

Therapists who had less well-established practices were forced to deal with managed care and had to join as many panels as possible to develop a client base. A few providers had left the practice, and many of those I interviewed had thought about leaving, or felt they might have to leave given the managed care environment:

> I'll try to decrease managed care, get out of managed care, find other niches, or get out of the field entirely. It's a noxious career with this much time invested in managed care activities. (Male MSW therapist)

BURNOUT IN THE PUBLIC SECTOR

> Managed care is a plan created to pretend to provide quality care and to be accountable. Anyone who has ever had to navigate a managed care system for their own care knows it has nothing to do with care. It has to do with mak-

ing money, laying on multiple levels of staff who monitor success (or prevent them) and destroying any bond you have with your consumers. (Nurse)

As noted previously, care has always been managed to some degree in public sector mental health, since reimbursements for care have been limited by legislative agencies. However, public sector mental health has also moved to an explicit managed care framework in which the treatment decisions made by providers are subject to various mechanisms of review. While an explicit system of managed care is fairly new to CARE, this study examines the ways in which it has changed the conditions of work and the providers' experience of burnout through a more quantitative examination of the survey data.

Managed care has the potential of reducing burnout in public sector organizations. Many providers at CARE in 1998 attributed burnout to the experience of "continuing to see the same clients forever" or "feeling that you see the same people admitted over and over again for the same thing and you wonder if we can really make a difference." One female case manager described burnout in the following terms:

> It's like having forty or so children and being the only "Mom" they have. It would help if the agency took on a role of promoting independence instead of dependence in clients.

For those who have worked with clients with severe and persistent mental illnesses, managed care may eventually help alleviate burnout by diffusing responsibility for treatment decisions and instilling clear criteria for difficult decisions about care. It may be very helpful for providers to have someone else make a determination that a given client is not going to make any progress, and should not continue in some program indefinitely. In short, public sector managed care may provide the kind of organizational supports and backup many providers identified as critical to alleviating burnout. Managed care may also force providers to work to develop natural community supports and to move clients through the system, hence eliminating the kind of dependency targeted by the provider quoted above.

However, the data collected in 2000 do not indicate that burnout is lessened with managed care. I concluded in Chapter 5 that providers at CARE also felt disillusioned with managed care and many were looking forward to retirement. The data from CARE analyzed in that chapter showed higher levels of burnout. Several providers commented that levels of burnout were higher, and noted the tremendous amount of turnover, especially among case managers. Providers were frustrated that treatment decisions were now being made on the basis of cost, rather than on clinical need and that cost was a higher priority than quality of care. Almost all of the providers gave feedback on the open-ended questions about the negative effect of cost-containment strategies on the quality of care, and the "devastating effect of shortened lengths of stay for chronically ill clients." A majority cited managed care as a significant source of stress, and felt that the increases in bureaucratic control over decisions had resulted in a lack of support from supervisors and administrators, and this was producing higher levels of burnout. One comment by a case manager seems to sum up the sentiments expressed about the sources of burnout:

> The contribution to burnout is frustration over the never-ending barriers and obstacles to the job created by the managed care system. It isn't the clients, or the staff so much as it's administration—who are out of touch with the work.

Almost one-half of the providers who completed the questionnaire cited concerns with the quality of care under managed care, and noted:

> Shortened length of stay in the hospital for the seriously mentally ill, resulting in clients' being sicker and sent into the community before they are stabilized. The community supports are not in place for our client population—housing and other resources. They just get sick, never stabilize, and return to the hospital. It's a revolving door. (Respondent #52)

With managed care, clinical staff had more administrative work and provided less direct client care. Providers report a twofold increase in time spent documenting care, and felt that efficiency was hindered by having all services certified by the review panel rather than the treatment team. The emphasis on cost was felt to interfere directly with client care, and clients were getting sicker and sicker. In response to a question about the problems with managed care one male case manager reported that

> fiscal issues are more important than client-related ones, there is a lack of information to ground level clinicians regarding changes, there is staff burnout—look at the number of new hires in case management over the past year. Case managers and other professionals seem to have to fight for services, our hard jobs are getting harder.

In terms of burnout and stress, providers at CARE overwhelming cited changes in the organization and lack of support for their work. The new management information system introduced with managed care and increased paperwork were cited by over one-half of the respondents as significant sources of stress. Burnout resulted "when client needs far outweigh what I (and the system) could provide" (#55); when "no matter how much you work you will never have met the expected need" (#77); "I am very burned out—it started with this job. I feel very hopeless about this job" (#78).

Almost every provider surveyed stated that a lack of support, mainly from supervisors but also from coworkers, was the major contributing factor to burnout. Closely related to the lack of support was the lack of decision-making input. These two factors were often mentioned in conjunction: "Not having input into decisions which impact my job and a lack of support from higher-level supervisors." Providers at CARE felt that their immediate team supervisors and clinical supervisors were great; higher-level management, where decisions about managed care and organizational restructuring were being made, targeted as the source of the problem. One case manager felt that "staff are not valued as important components of the agency, only as people meeting a need, whatever meeting that need will cost the employee." In other words, care work had become a commodity. Burnout could be alleviated by more organizational supports and incentives, and a greater focus on client care that "stop[ped] viewing the clients as numerical data" (#77). One provider (#75) stated that CARE "needed to focus on the needs of clients, not on the desires of the insurance company. They need to stop putting up hoops to jump through."

The survey data allow for some quantitative consideration of the relationship between organizational working conditions, feelings about work, emotional labor, and burnout. In addition to the indicators of working conditions presented in Chapter 5, I also created an index of emotional labor. Providers were asked how often on a scale of *never* to almost *always* they (1) had to work with clients to establish a relationship; (2) work with clients on many different aspects of their lives; (3) understand what my clients are feeling; (4) understand the unique needs of my clients. This index could go from 0 (no emotional labor) to 12. Of the 45 providers who answered these questions, only 33.3 percent had levels below 10. Forty percent had a score of 12 (the highest level of emotional labor possible). The overall mean was 10.27 with a standard deviation of 1.84. In addition to an index (and additive in nature) the emotional labor measure also had good scale properties, with a reliability of .7075, indicating that the measures of emotional labor are highly interrelated. Emotional labor was significantly higher for women. A second measure of emotional labor is the percentage of time spent in direct client contact (excluding phone calls). Providers reported spending close to one-half of their time in direct client contact (49.55 percent with a standard deviation of 25.28).

I also examined responses toward managed care by looking at how often the financial mechanisms to manage care resulted in (1) reduced use of community services; (2) reduced duration of treatment; (3) provision of less intensive services than you would have recommended; (4) a greater reliance on medication and (5) reduced lengths of stay. This scale could go from 0 to 10 (never to almost always). Forty-four respondents completed these questions, and 15 percent were under 5, 43.2 percent were from 5 to 7, and 42 percent had scores above 7, indicating that perceptions about the negative effects of managed care on the quality of care were pervasive. The mean was 6.68 with a standard deviation of 2.62.

The questionnaire also provides information on goal incongruence, the degree to which providers felt that current organizational goals and practices varied from what they thought the organization ought to be doing. Client-level goals (more outreach, high technical quality, improve client functioning, client satisfaction, client's families satisfaction, and protection of the community from violent and unwanted behavior, improve the quality of the client's life) and organizational goals (contain costs, enhance revenues, satisfy staff, innovate, collaborate between agencies, expand service offerings, integrate services to diverse client populations) were evaluated. Respondents are asked to indicate a percentage (0–100) for how important they think a goal currently is for the organization, and another percentage for how important they think the goal ought to be. Current goals are subtracted from ideal goals in order to arrive at a goal incongruence score. Higher numbers indicate providers thought a goal should be more important than it was; negative numbers indicate the organization places too much emphasis on a given goal. Table 9 examines changes in the degree of goal incongruence between 1998 and 2000. The overall goal incongruence

Table 9. Goal Incongruence[a]
Mean Percentage and (s.d.)

Organizational Goals	1998	2000	p-value
Reach Out to More Clients	15.0 (22.97)	18.78 (26.04)	.460
High Technical Quality	27.79 (24.64)	21.46 (32.31)	.301
Improved Client Functioning	20.94 (18.95)	23.95 (23.84)	.501
Client Satisfaction	13.87 (22.66)	23.26 (29.51)	.089
Satisfaction of Client's Families	13.33 (20.03)	20.71 (29.51)	.132
Protect Community from Violent/Unwanted Behavior	16.80 (25.52)	19.52 (25.15)	.600
Improve Quality of Client's Life	22.91 (23.96)	28.17 (18.07)	.343
Contain Costs	−4.55 (23.73)	−9.88 (24.77)	.006
Enhance Revenues	−9.77 (29.27)	−8.95 (28.29)	.003
Satisfied Staff	40.95 (33.32)	45.24 (26.27)	.506
Innovate	32.95 (26.35)	31.30 (34.41)	.793
Improve Interorganizational Relations	30.42 (28.18)	34.41 (29.48)	.513
Expand Service Offerings	20.31 (23.76)	29.53 (25.74)	.081
Integrate Service Offerings to Diverse Client Populations	19.89 (25.89)	27.14 (29.57)	.219

[a]A higher number indicates providers thought the goal should be more important than it currently was; a negative number indicates they thought the organization placed too much emphasis on a given goal.

score is 21.97 in 2001; it was 20.35 in 1998, and while there is no significant difference in the two periods, there are in fact significant changes in the levels of goal incongruence for individual goals. Providers felt that more emphasis needed to be placed on satisfying the clients and their families, and on improving the quality of the client's life. They felt that too much emphasis was being placed on containing costs and enhancing revenue, and that more emphasis should be placed on satisfying staff, expanding service offerings, and integrating services.

Important to the effective management of labor is autonomy and a good working environment. In terms of the working environment, one scale, satisfaction with operating procedures, actually measures the degree to which providers find their work subject to bureaucratic control. Higher levels of bureaucratic constraint indicated agreement that (1) many of our rules and procedures are making doing a good job difficult; (2) my efforts to do a good job are blocked by red tape; (3) I have too much paperwork to do; (4) I have too much work to do. This scale is also an indicator of the "speed-up" process in which providers are given more work than they can do. A lower score (from 1 to 5) indicates greater dissatisfaction with bureaucratic control, and the mean was 2.65. While dissatisfaction with operating procedures was higher in 2000, it was not significantly different from that in 1998 (before managed care).

A second measure of providers' relationship with their work is satisfaction with the nature of work, which is indicated by response to the questions (1) I sometimes feel my job is meaningless; (2) I like doing the things I do at work; (3) I feel a sense of pride in my work; (4) my job is enjoyable. Levels of satisfaction with the nature of the work were significantly lower in 2000 (dropping from 3.99 to 3.65 on a five point scale). Similarly, levels of autonomy were also significantly lower in 2000 (dropping from 3.56 to 3.3 on a five point scale). The questions to measure autonomy capture provider's degree of control over decisions about client care.

1. I feel that I am supervised more closely than is necessary.
2. I feel that I have sufficient input into the program of care for each of my clients.
3. I am sometimes frustrated because all my activities seem programmed for me.
4. I am sometimes required to do things on my job that are against my better professional judgment.
5. I have too much responsibility and not enough authority.

I focus on two dimensions of burnout: emotional exhaustion and depersonalization. The third dimension of burnout, a lack of personal accomplishment, can also be attributed to a lack of professional recognition as well as burnout. Emotional exhaustion and depersonalization are more clearly tied to work with clients and to the performance of emotional labor. Levels of both indicators of burnout were relatively low; emotional exhaustion was 2.42 on a six-point scale and depersonalization was .92 on a six-point scale. Levels of emotional exhaustion had significantly increased since 1998 (from 1.86 to 2.42).

Indicators of Emotional Exhaustion
I feel drained from my work.
I feel used up at the end of the workday.
I feel fatigued when I get up in the morning and have to face another day
    on the job.
Working with people all day is really a strain for me.
I feel burned out from my job.
I feel frustrated by my job.

Indicators of Depersonalization
I feel I treat some clients as if they were impersonal objects.
I've become more callous toward people since I took this job.
I worry that this job is hardening me emotionally.
I don't really care what happens to some clients.
I feel clients blame me for some of their problems.

While the numbers are small, a causal examination of the factors that predict negative attitudes toward managed care and burnout yield some interesting findings. An examination of the correlations between the indices of psychological burnout (emotional exhaustion and a sense of depersonalization) shows that burnout is significantly associated with bureaucratic control (increased paperwork and rules), a lack of satisfaction with the nature of work (or feeling work is meaningless and lacking pride in work), and decreased job autonomy and critical attitudes toward the cost-containment emphasis of managed care (Table 10). Emotional exhaustion is also significantly related to decreased (not increased) client contact. Emotional labor is not related to burnout, although it negatively related to autonomy and positively related to goal incongruence. Goal incongruence is associated with greater dissatisfaction with the organization, work, and lower levels of autonomy. Critical views of managed care are also associated with dissatisfaction with the organization, lower levels of autonomy, goal incongruence, and higher levels of emotional labor, indicating that managed care is having an impact on providers' ability to do their work in a manner they consider meaningful.

Table 11 is an Ordinary Least Squares regression analysis of burnout, which shows that autonomy and goal incongruence are significant predictors of emotional exhaustion, and that critical attitudes toward managed care approaches statistical significance (especially given the small sample

Table 10. Correlations Among Key Organizational Variables, Emotional Labor and Burnout (all correlations above .20 are significant at 0.10 level). N=35

	(1)	(2)	(3)	(4)	(5)	(6)	(7)	(8)
1. Emotional Exhaustion	1.0							
2. Depersonalization	.695							
3. Satisfied with Bureaucracy	−.723	−.377						
4. Satisfied with Work	−.393	−.442	.426					
5. Autonomy	−.732	−.431	.817	.414				
6. % Direct Client Care	−.444	−.148	.402	.175	.326			
7. Goal Incongruence	.166	−.036	−.449	−.294	−.431	−.039		
8. Emotional Labor	.034	−.044	.036	−.072	−.276	.091	.249	
9. Critical of Managed Care	.222	.052	−.307	−.017	−.286	.170	.486	.350

size). Providers who have less autonomy, higher levels of dissatisfaction with organizational goals, and who are critical of managed care are more likely to experience emotional exhaustion. Goal incongruence and dissatisfaction with the nature of work are significant predictors of depersonalization. This analysis shows that it is not emotional labor per se, or bureaucracy and client demands, but the feeling that the organization is not meeting professionally based criteria for care, which is the source of burnout.

Burnout results when providers are prevented from fulfilling their therapeutic roles in the manner they considered viable, when they "lacked control," and so providers subject to managed care at CARE are experiencing the same kind of disillusionment as those in private practice. A good number of providers at CARE responded to my question about how they

Table 11. Causal Analysis of Burnout Under Managed Care (Standardized coefficients, standard error, and p-value)

Independent Variables	Emotional Exhaustion			Depersonalization		
	Beta	s.e.	p-value	Beta	s.e.	p-value
Satisfied With Bureaucracy	−.214	.442	.391	.095	.389	.782
Satisfied With Work	−.136	.250	.288	−.389	.220	.033
Autonomy	−.524	.463	.029	−.517	.407	.111
% Client Contact	−.201	.007	.125	.026	.006	.883
Goal Incongruence	−.281	.014	.052	−.362	.012	.068
Emotional Labor	−.098	.130	.499	−.187	.115	.353
Critical of Managed Care	.210	.077	.155	.163	.068	.418
R-Square	.678		.000	.385		.047

thought their work would change in the next ten years with the same kind of admission made by many of those in private practice: "I'm going to retire and escape this mess."

OVERBURDENED PROVIDERS: IMPLICATIONS FOR BURNOUT

I have argued that burnout results when the emotional labor of providers is curtailed to such a degree that they are not able to perform their clinical role in a professional and personally appropriate manner, and their professional identity is not confirmed or enhanced. Providers need autonomy or control over their work role, and managed care seeks to reduce this professional prerogative. As a result, burnout is exacerbated under managed care. Edwards (1997: 205) describes the effect that managed care had on her sense of work identity following an argument with a managed care company about the care she had recommended for a client.

> I was certainly aware that the telephone call had left me anxious, depressed, and angry. I felt demeaned, powerless, and doubtful of my own competence. I was aware of a sense of having failed the patient and of some barely perceived fear with regard to her response . . . My self-confidence was also diminished by the presence of an unknown, unseen overseer with the power to make the most fundamental decisions about treatment . . . Despite my many years of training and experience, I was forced to confront the fact that I was no longer appropriately in charge of my clinical practice.

The majority of private practice providers I interviewed had undergone the same kind of professional and personal demoralization in dealing with managed care companies. The aspect of their jobs private practice clinicians most disliked was dealing with managed care, or having to deal with the additional paperwork required by managed care. Not only were the bureaucratic requirements frustrating and time-consuming, they also interfered with care and prevented clients from receiving the kind of care providers felt was appropriate. Thus managed care was a significant source of stress:

> I feel stressed when I have managed care-giving three sessions for an update and delaying payment or denying care due to their mistakes. I am also stressed when managed care cuts fees or refuses to cover the costs of the licenses they require. (Female MSW therapist)

Yet such bureaucratic hassles did not produce burnout. Burnout resulted when the provider felt "a lack of energy, depressed, helpless, angry about those institutions which interfered with the client's care and health."

Burnout was a consequence of dealing with "the other client—insurance companies and the feelings of helplessness when professionals were not treated as professionals." Burnout was seen a form of dehumanization, or alienation from one's life calling. The commodification of care was directly responsible:

> Our society has defined success in recent times by productivity and numbers—a bottom-line mentality which is often opposed to the therapeutic process and dehumanizes the clinician as well as the client. (Male therapist)

Providers at CARE targeted much of their frustration against top-level managers whom they perceived as being responsible for the managed care framework. Providers at CARE were also deeply concerned about the quality of the care received by their clients and denials for needed services. They experienced a sense of dismay as the gains that had been made during the years of community mental health were being lost. As one nurse lamented:

> Almost everything I used to do in this job was important. I had a great relationship with consumers assigned to my caseload, I have worked front line for almost twenty years. I have been recognized by individuals and organizations for my advocacy on behalf of mentally ill consumers. With the changes in Medicaid and the introduction of this case management system, all of this has changed. I got into this profession because I like consumers and their families. I'm good at what I do and I make a real different in folks' lives. With the death of a real community support system, I worry what is to become of our consumers. Why can't people learn from what works? Now we are going backwards. We are doomed to repeat our mistakes.

In conclusion, burnout is a likely consequence when the organization limits the emotional labor of providers. I predict that managed care will exacerbate burnout in two ways. First, by seeking to specify the type of treatment model or role the provider is to assume with a client, managed care seeks to change the work identity of providers. As described in Chapter 3, providers have been socialized into a model of care that emphasizes long-term continuous care and the provision of supports for clients with severe mental illnesses. Yet managed care emphasizes short-term, brief, focused, results-oriented therapy. Second, since cost-containment is likely to further reduce resources, providers will experience an exacerbated speed-up of multiple demands and have too many clients. The speed-up provides an organizational context likely to produce not only increased stress but burnout as well, because the provider is prevented from meeting professionally prescribed feeling rules.

8 Shifting Institutional Contexts for Mental Health Care

This chapter examines new and emerging institutional forces that will shape mental health care in the coming years. As I argued in Chapter 1, the institutional environment has a direct bearing on mental health care. The institutional environment consists of beliefs about mental health and illness, social preferences for quality care and cost-containment, and professional norms and practices. Mental health care organizations and providers must conform to these various institutional beliefs and demands in order to maintain legitimacy and survive. However, these institutional demands can be contradictory and ambiguous. In particular, there is conflict between the professionally based logics of community care and the institutional logic of commodification and cost-containment. As Shore and Beigel (1996: 77) argue, managed care represents a "controversial" challenge to "traditional definitions of mental illness and treatment goals." In this chapter I identify and describe the key forces and organizations that exert various forms of institutional pressure on mental health care systems. In particular, I look for evidence of countervailing power, or forces that limit managed care's potential for abuse.

COMMODIFICATION AND CONTRADICTION

Light (1997) describes four types of health care system: the community, professional, state (or sponsor-based), and the corporate. Each system is distinguished by a different set of values, or institutional logic. The primary goal in a state-sponsored health system is a healthy population (which benefits the state); a professionally driven system seeks to provide quality care to everyone who needs it; a community-based system addresses chronic health problems and seeks to minimize disease and death via preventive measures. The corporate model, which currently dominates, is characterized by the desire to increase market share and maximize profits (Light 1997). The commodification of health care is the movement from a provider- to a buyer-driven system of care, and was a result of the "buyers' revolt" due to escalating health care costs in the 1970s and 1980s. Scott et al. (2000) describe the increased reliance on market control in health care as the era of managerial control and market mechanisms, dating from 1983 to the present. The earlier eras of health care placed primary value on healthcare quality (era of professional dominance) or building comprehensive community health systems and insuring access for all (era of federal dominance). The new institutional environment emphasizes cost-containment and efficiency. Market controls replace professional associations and regulatory controls as the primary means of governance while health care corporations replace independent physicians and the government as the key institutional actors.

Meyer (1990) provides us with a more generalized model of commodification. The commodity model arises from the work of economists and is based upon the idea that current environmental pressures favor market solutions. Because inefficiencies can result from rationalized organizational structures (i.e., bureaucracy), new organizational forms are governed by financial controls that are assumed to lead to desired outcomes and behaviors. Consequently, efficiency is not an outcome of organization structure. Instead, organizational structures are the outcomes of efficiency constraints. In the case of health care, managed health care organizations and corporate players have the tools to maximize efficiency outcomes, and health care has become a commodity. Health care providers have lost power, and their work is being increasingly subject to efficiency criteria. At this point, there is clear conflict between professional logics of care and the demands for efficiency and cost-containment (which I have referred to as the logic of commodification). The empirical question is whether professional logics will change to incorporate efficiency demands or be engulfed by the institutional logic of commodification. However, the larger conflict inherent in the commodification of care has to do with the imposition of efficiency constraints on organizations that operate in institutional environments.

One of the central tenets of institutional theory is that organizations operating in institutional environments must conform to wider normative standards rather than technically driven considerations of efficiency. With regard to mental health care, the wider normative standards have been determined largely by mental health professionals who, by both personal inclination and professional socialization, are primarily concerned with providing quality care to as many clients as possible (hence meeting the goals of both access and quality care). Because mental health care, and mental health care outcomes, cannot be easily measured or achieved with known technologies, legitimacy was attained in the past by providers' meeting institutional expectations about what constitutes appropriate clinical practice (Cook and Wright 1995). The conflict between professionally generated standards for mental health care and technical criteria for efficiency was resolved by various means of protecting the technical core of mental health care work from outside evaluation (Scheid-Cook 1990). However, managed care insists that providers' furnish empirical evidence of effective treatment and cost-savings, and seeks direct control over their work. How have providers responded?

First, the providers have acknowledged the conflict between professional and bureaucratic standards of care. Minkoff (1997: 13) describes the concern among providers about "the perceived incompatibility of managed care with community mental health ideology, and with their own deeply held principles and ideals regarding public sector service." However, he calls upon providers to try to resolve this incongruence. Ogles et al. (1998: 255) argue that "the managed care emphasis on appropriate care in fact matches nicely with the system-of-care value of community-based care." In particular, managed care emphasizes care in the least restrictive setting (outpatient versus hospital, home versus institutional living). Managed care may also allow for investment of profits into system development, and for the coordination of diverse funding streams (ibid.).

One of the early documents that provided guidelines for developing managed care systems of care for those with serious mental illness was the Bazelon Center for Mental Health Law manual, *Managing Managed Care for Publicly Financed Mental Health Services* (1995). The authors began with the premise that the needs of clients in the public sector were different from those in the private sector, and that these individuals required a "range of rehabilitation and support services not commonly covered by traditional insurance" (ibid.: 9). In order to meet the needs of these clients, managed care plans must offer rehabilitation, case management, assertive community treatment, consumer-controlled alternatives, and "other services necessary to achieve positive outcomes" (ibid.: 20). In addition, the managed care system must also guarantee access and remove barriers to access. Yet these outcomes are defined in terms of professional models of care rather than in terms of the commodity model that actually governs managed care entities.

The conflict between cost-containment and care was recognized, and the Bazelon Center (ibid.: 31) advised against a full risk system (i.e., pre-negotiated capitation) because of "managed care's inherent incentive to reduce services." Furthermore, outcomes should contain measures of quality, such as client satisfaction and quality of life. In addition, while the role of the state would be reduced in managed systems, the state should serve as a watchdog, and establish standards to protect consumers. Specifically the Bazelon Center (ibid.: 36) recommends:

1. Precertification and utilization review should be conducted by trained, professional staff who do not have a stake in denying care.
2. Review criteria should be well-defined and clearly understood by providers, and should be available to the public.
3. Rapid access to emergency care should be available without time-consuming preapproval.

More recent responses to managed care also reflect the inclination of professionals to work within the framework imposed by managed care, rather than challenge the system itself (Minkoff and Pollack 1997: xi–xii).

> We and our colleagues may feel disoriented, frightened, insecure, angry, and discouraged. Yet we can't give up. We remain committed to improving the care for people we have traditionally served . . . We feel the best response to the managed care revolution is to involve ourselves in the planning and implementation of services so that our clients are protected and that the public mental health principles that we feel most strongly about are incorporated into the newly developed systems of care.

Minkoff (1997: 21) views the ideology of managed care as "strikingly similar to the original ideology of the community mental health movement." He articulates a Public Sector Managed Care (PSMC) ideology that fuses the ideologies of community-based care and managed care. The PSMC principals are as follows (Minkoff 1997: 19):

1. The needs of an entire community, as defined by the public sector payer, should be addressed.
2. Services should be accessible to the entire population, not just those with serious mental illnesses.
3. Systems-of-care should be organized to provide comprehensive, continuous, efficient and cost-effective services.
4. Interventions should be targeted to enhance reliance on consumer empowerment and client strengths rather than fostering overdependence on professional care.
5. Triage systems should offer comprehensive community-based alternatives to inpatient care.
6. Per capita rates will encourage providers to manage resources efficiently and to evaluate resource needs through outcome evaluation.
7. The elimination of a two-tiered system of care (public versus private) by funding private providers to provide care for public clients, and funding public providers to develop services that can compete for private dollars.

It is clear that this integrated ideology is an ideal typification in which care-based principles are *theoretically* combined with demands for cost-containment and efficiency. Yet there is no inherent expectation that a system should provide for the full continuum of care if this is not deemed cost-efficient. Minkoff (1997) recognizes this, and argues that there are a number of critical questions that need to be answered in order for the principles of community-based care to be safeguarded. First, who makes the ultimate decisions about cost versus quality? Are there external means to monitor quality? Is there some community-based control? How is the conflict between focused, brief therapy, and long-term care resolved? These questions all go to the root of the contradictions between managed care and community-based treatment ideologies.

CARE has sought to provide the kind of system envisioned by Minkoff (1977), and to maintain professional control within a managed care framework. Yet, as shown in Chapter 5, CARE's restructuring efforts were in large part a response to efficiency demands from the state government. In particular, CARE sought to develop its own managed care plan before state mandated managed care. In the late 1990s, there was widespread belief in a move to privatize mental health care services. More specifically, it was believed that the state would select a for-profit managed care firm to manage care for all of the state mental health care programs. Administrators at CARE felt that they would not be able to maintain their system of care under external control, and they sought to develop a model system of care that could be used throughout the state.

In implementing managed care, CARE consciously sought to preserve the goals of community-based, integrated care. It has sought to make the public sector population eligible for services and to make services accessible to the entire population, not just those with serious mental illness. CARE has retained the core elements of a comprehensive system of services developed over the past decades, and has sought to extend and improve on that system. Finally, CARE is on its way to eliminating the two-tiered system of care by funding private providers to take on public clients, and funding public providers to develop services that can compete for private dollars. CARE is a good example of how managed care is blurring the distinction between private and public mental health care (Minkoff and Pollack 1997).

Despite the ideological commitment to comprehensive, continuous care, there has been a great deal of conflict over the emphasis on short-term treatment associated with cost-containment and managed care, and the longer-term treatment and social supports associated with community-based care. The organizational changes made at CARE (the new triage system, new organization of case management teams, and the new divisions for utilization review) all ensure that clients get more short-term treatment. These changes are all in response to efficiency demands. At the same time, CARE has also responded to larger demands for quality care, and is one of the first public sector mental health care agencies to apply (and receive provisional approval) for national accreditation for quality care. In fact, a growing concern with ensuring quality care is an institutional demand that may have the power to check the excesses of demands for cost-containment. As noted by Mechanic and McAlpine (1999: 17) "until we have (and use) more sophisticated quality measurement, the temptation will remain to manage costs and not care."

SAFEGUARDING QUALITY CARE

Campbell et al. (2000) define quality of care in terms of two principal dimensions: access and effectiveness. Do patients get the care they need, and is the care effective when they get it? Effectiveness of care includes both clinical effectiveness (i.e., the treatment reduced or eliminated the symptoms) and interpersonal relationships (patient's satisfaction with provider). A number of groups have sought to safeguard standards of quality and access in the face of managed care's bottom line of cost-containment. Responding to pressures to establish a set of standards to protect the quality of care, in 1996 the Institute of Medicine formed the Committee on Quality Assurance and Accreditation Guidelines for Managed Behavioral Health Care. The committee's mission was to "develop a framework to guide the development, use, and evaluation of performance indicators, accreditation standards, and quality improvement mechanisms" (Institute of Medicine 1997: v). In terms of mental health care, the Institute found a great deal of fragmentation as well as variability from state to state. In terms of outcomes, the Institute noted lack of consensus over what constitutes successful treatment and called for more research in order to develop standards for mental health care (ibid.). The National Association for Healthcare Quality (NAHQ) is another organization that seeks to improve the quality of care given to individuals in managed care organizations by establishing standards. Further, the NAHQ also promotes the development of healthcare professionals.

However, quality continues to remain a concern (Institute of Medicine 2001). Scanlon et al. (2000) examined the degree to which managed care organizations have responded to external pressures for quality. Six managed care plans in four states were selected (the sample was not random) and CEOs, medical directors, and quality improvement directors were interviewed by telephone. Scanlon et al. did find strong incentives for quality improvement (QI); most managed care organizations have QI departments. However, there was little evidence that managed care plans had structures in place to ensure that their provider networks met QI demands.

The controversy over both the definition and the treatment of mental health has led to debates over how to measure mental health outcomes (Horwitz 2002; Mirowsky and Ross 2002). Despite these more theoretical debates, a body of services literature has identified mental health outcomes (for a review of major texts see Salzer 1999). For the most part, these measures reflect the emphasis on evidence-based practice with little regard for quality (MacFarland 2001). Subsequently, the Agency for Healthcare Research and Quality, the National Institute of Mental Health, and the Substance Abuse, Mental Health and Services Administration funded research to assess current mental health measures and to develop a National Inventory of Mental Health Quality Measures (Herman et al. 2000).

Researchers identified eighty-six measures for mental health and identified various domains that assess quality (ibid.). The study was limited to those measures associated with clinical and administrative processes (as opposed to outcome). The quality domains identified, and the degree to which these domains are reflected by organizations for the assessment of the quality of mental health care include: treatment appropriateness (65 percent), continuity (26 percent), access (26 percent), coordination (13 percent), detection (12 percent) and prevention (6 percent). Based on this research, an inventory of mental health measures has been developed and is available on the internet at the Center for Quality Assessment and Improvement in Mental Health (2003). Over three hundred process measures are included, and they reflect seven domains of quality (access, assessment, treatment, continuity, coordination, patient safety, and prevention).

In 2000 CARE began working to obtain National Committee for Quality Assurance accreditation and developed a QI committee whose function was to ensure that outcomes were consistent with mandated standards for quality care. Outcome targets were specified for each of the major divisions providing care to clients. Partial hospitalization and crisis stabilization simply report the number of hospitalizations averted, which Herman (2000) argues is a process measure rather than an outcome measure. The outcome targets of the other major divisions are as follows:

Adult Case Management
1. 85 percent of consumers will have decreased frequency of crisis episodes (measured by reduced rate on inpatient hospitalizations).
2. 25 percent of consumers who receive case management will achieve or maintain independent living.
3. 4 percent of consumers who receive case management will be engaged in competitive employment.
4. 20 percent of consumers who receive case management will be engaged in prevocational training, volunteer work, school, or intermittent odd jobs.

Clubhouses
1. 10 percent of consumers in clubhouse will be successfully engaged in part-time or full-time competitive employment each quarter.

2. 35 percent of clubhouse consumers are engaged in volunteer, school, or vocational training.
3. Consumers engaged in clubhouse services will demonstrate a reduction in inpatient hospitalization when compared to overall division rates of hospitalization.

Medical Services
1. 75 percent of consumers receiving medication education during the quarter are compliant.
2. 85 percent decrease in the frequency of crisis episodes for consumers in medical services (those clients who are receiving medication only).
3. 90 percent of consumers surveyed by Medical Services are satisfied with their services.

These targets (or goals) are consistent with the basic objectives of community care: to avert hospitalization and to allow for some return to independent life and employment. In the past, CARE had measured outcomes in terms of service-level acuity (overall level of functioning). Tracking client outcomes consisted of examining changes in aggregate levels of service-level acuity with no attempt to measure changes at the individual level or to set targets. Improvements in service-level acuity are no longer assessed, and outcomes are still specified at the aggregate level (i.e., we do not know how many patients actually improve). Division supervisors report quarterly on these outcomes, providing specific data to demonstrate that for the most part they meet their outcome targets.

As part of the QI process, patient records are reviewed each quarter by a separate division, which assesses the appropriateness of treatment in terms of the following specific indicators:

1. Clinical accuracy based on assessment information and client's level of functioning.
2. Service plan reflects the strengths and needs of the consumer as indicated in the referral assessment or case manager assessment.
3. Service plan includes short-term measurable goals that are behavior specific.
4. Periodic reviews of the service plan justify continuing services.
5. Service plan reflects family/collateral involvement.
6. The frequency of contact is adequate to address the acuity/clinical needs of the consumer.

Quality improvement reports indicated that divisions do meet these indicators of quality. However, these outcomes and QI standards reflect an emphasis on efficiency, rather than on professionally mandated standards of care. There is an obvious emphasis on short-term treatment and medication compliance. Quality of care is measured in terms of treatment appropriateness, with little attention paid to continuity or access. We do not know if those who are receiving medication services alone are in fact stable in the community, nor does any follow-up of discharged patients ensure that they are still doing well. While the basics of community care are evident, there is a strong emphasis on efficiency.

CARE has received provisional accreditation as a Managed Behavioral Healthcare Organization (MBHO) from the NCQA, and it is the first governmental MBHO in the country to obtain this accreditation. It has almost completed the process of moving from a public sector service provider, to a manager of services. This is in response to state-level mandated legislative changes that constitute the most systematic reform to the mental health system since the development of the community catchment area system. I turn to a consideration of this major institutional demand.

STATE-MANDATED PRIVATIZATION

Throughout the 1990s, states and counties placed various components of their community care systems under managed care (Croze 2000). Most public sector mental health care is paid for by Medicaid dollars, and the proportion of Medicaid enrollees enrolled in managed care plans increased substantially in the 1990s. However, the level of Medicaid managed care penetration varies widely from state to state as does the way in which managed care operates (Hanson and Huskamp 2001). Some states use integrated programs where the state Medicaid agency contracts with managed care organizations to provide both physical and mental health (or behavioral health) services, while others carve out mental health services. Some states use fee-for-service programs but exclude mental health from their Medicaid managed care (ibid.). While a great deal of information about various state Medicaid managed care programs exists, "relatively little is known about how different types of programs may influence the quality of mental health and substance abuse services" (ibid.: 449). Part of the problem in assessing different approaches lies in the tremendous variability at both the state and local levels. This variability also raises serious concerns about equity of care (Hanson and Huskamp 2001). The Bazelon Center (2000) has published a report on state's Medicaid reforms entitled "Effective Public Management of Mental Health Care: Views from States on Medicaid Reforms That Enhance Service Integration and Accountability." The report showed a great deal of variability from state to state in their use of managed care, and described the problems in seeking to privatize public mental health systems. A more recent report (Bazelon 2001) also describes problems with state mental health reforms.

In terms of research on state efforts to privatize mental health services, Fendell (1998) studied two managed care organizations that ran the state's mental health services. He found that these firms distorted care decisions to meet bottom-line goals and the state was unable to monitor the client outcomes as the companies controlled the data. Strout (1998) also raises important questions about statewide carve-outs in Iowa where only services that met the criteria of medical necessity were authorized, and clients with serious mental illnesses were not getting the community supports they needed. In addition, inpatient care was denied and clients reported problems gaining access to the new system (ibid.). The Bazelon Center (2000, 2001) also found that in many states privatized managed care resulted in fewer services to those with serious mental illnesses and neglect of rehabilitative care.

Despite these troubling signs of its failure to provide for those with serious mental illnesses, North Carolina decided to mandate managed care. North Carolina's mental health services are combined with developmental disabilities and substance abuse services; consequently both the state division and each area authority have the title of Department (or Division) of Mental Health, Developmental Disabilities, and Substance Abuse Services (MH, DD, SA). Catchments are defined along county lines, and most of the current thirty-nine area programs in North Carolina include two or more counties. Only two programs are single-county area authorities. Consequently, area authorities must not only provide care for diverse treatment populations (i.e., MH, DD, SA), they must also provide that care within the context of considerable county and regional variation. While the largest group of clients are those with mental health needs, close to one-half of the 2000 state MH/DD/SA budget went for developmental disabilities. While the three communities do work together to gain resources via a joint advocacy coalition, there is considerable conflict over scarce resources.

North Carolina moved to review its mental health system and make needed reforms fairly late compared to other states. This gave them the advantage of learning from the system's failures and, it is hoped, duplicate its best practices. The reform was in response to a growing mental health crisis due to rapid growth in expenditures for developmental disabilities, growing fiscal problems of community mental health centers (local authorities), and problems with misuse of federal Medicaid dollars.[1] There was also a crisis of leadership both within the State Division of MH, DD, SA, and within the legislature. In addition, the *Charlotte Observer* ran a series exposing neglect in the state mental health system. In short, the mental health system suffered from a legitimacy crisis.

In 1998 the State Auditor was charged with overseeing a comprehensive study of the state's psychiatric hospitals and mental health delivery system. The loss in confidence in the State Division of MH, DD, and SA was so severe that no one trusted the agency to conduct its own research on the system of care. Consequently, two private consulting firms were hired and a final report was made to the State Auditor in 2000. This report made specific recommendations for system-wide reform. In response to the crisis the state legislature named the Legislative Oversight Committee in 2000 to refine and implement the redesign plan. This committee developed legislation (HB 381/SB 374), which mandates major reform to the state-wide system of care, and the legislation passed in 2002, with implementation beginning July 1, 2003. There was broad-based input into the various drafts of the legislation. Most area programs were against the changes but the Oversight Committee perceived that consumers and advocates for the most part supported the plan.

Mental health services will no longer be provided by local authorities; instead, agencies will contract out all direct care services through a qualified provider network. Public sector mental health will cease to exist in North Carolina. The major features of the system reform are as follows:

1. The downsizing of hospitals from four to three and the reduction of bed capacity (except in the Western region of the state where bed capacity is to be expanded).
2. The area Authorities operate as managed behavioral healthcare organizations. Each local authority develops a business plan (which must be approved) to become a Local Management Entity (LME) spelling out how local authorities will manage (rather than provide) services. LMEs can contract out management, or they can manage services themselves. LMEs must also obtain national certification.
3. The renovation and expansion of substance abuse treatment.
4. The creation of uniform portals of entry, with a statewide system contractor to provide referral, crisis hotline and utilization management.
5. The development of integrated payment and management systems.
6. The development of a competency-based system for providers.
7. The development of an Office of Consumer Affairs at the state level and mandated consumer involvement at the local level.

Most fundamentally, the reform targets services to those with the most serious illnesses as defined by psychiatric diagnoses and Global Assessment of Functioning levels. Within this target population six priority groups are identified: those with multiple diagnoses, those who are homeless, those in the criminal justice system, those who are elderly, those who are deaf, and minorities. Two target groups are also defined for children: those with development disabilities and those with substance abuse problems. Local authorities have been given three years (beginning July 1, 2003) to implement their local business plans and to complete systemwide reforms.

We will examine how CARE has responded both to the state-mandated reform and to the response of a nearby three county system. CARE began its movement to managed care five years ago, and at the time of the mandate was already managing services and had developed all of the mechanisms to manage care. In fact, at one time CARE asked the state for permission to manage services for all area programs in the state. CARE had been cited by state officials as a model system and had already received provisional accreditation from the National Committee for Quality Assurance. Furthermore, CARE had been contracting out more and more of its services to private agencies, and had planned to outsource the few remaining service functions. The state plan allows local authorities to continue to provide core services such as crises assistance and emergency care. In short, CARE has already met most of the standards set by the state.

As are other area authorities, CARE is most concerned with the limits imposed on its services to target populations. According to the state plan, area authorities can continue to provide "core" services (screening, assessment, emergencies services and triage, care coordination, consultation, education, and prevention) to all county residents. However, these services must be brief and are to be directed at linking consumers to community-based supports. There is concern among providers that many who need care will not receive it under new state targets. This fear in compounded by the fact that as of July 1, 2003, the state had not set a budget for local authorities to work with. Undoubtedly, service provision will be constrained by funding limitations.

In contrast to CARE, New Directions (also a pseudonym) had a great deal of work to do to prepare its business plan. New Directions has been a full-service provider for three counties in a rural part of North Carolina. They elected to become a manager of care (following CARE's model) but had to determine which services should be kept and which should be outsourced and privatized within the three-year window. In 2000 New Directions hired a consultant and began a two-year process of developing the framework for a new system of care. Of course, the expenses of this development are not reimbursable! They had to reorganize its management structure completely and develop mechanisms for evaluation and quality improvement as well as utilization review. They drafted a continuous quality improvement plan and measures of effectiveness (access, quality of care, administrative processes, consumer outcomes). The organization will have to seek national accreditation in 2004 and are considering the NCQA.

New Directions' three-year plan allows for the gradual privatization of direct care services, and they have developed a Qualified Provider Network. In addition, they have created a database of community organizations that can meet the needs of nontarget populations. Because New Directions is concerned about the needs of these nontarget consumers, they will develop a system to track referrals and the availability of services. In addition, they have arranged for a long-term evaluation of their managed care system.[2] While not happy about the reforms, or the new system of care, providers at New Directions remain committed to offering quality care, recovery, and empowerment to the consumer. Consumers have been given major roles both in designing the new system of care and in serving as its key leaders. While the state mandated greater consumer involvement, many area authorities hand-picked their consumer advocates. New Directions actively sought broad-based input from consumers in the community (not just those in current advocacy positions or receiving services). The ideology of consumer empowerment and recovery is another institutional demand that may play an important role in the future of mental health care. Sabin and Daniels (2001) argue that a stronger consumer presence (with some power) can make managed care more accountable.

ADVOCACY AS COUNTERVAILING POWER

The major advocacy group seeking to guarantee care to those with severe mental illnesses is the National Alliance for the Mentally Ill (NAMI). Currently NAMI has 220,000 members and their web site is an excellent resource for consumers and advocates. The website (www.nami.org) contains recent treatment news, a link to the President's Commission on Mental Health report (released in the summer of 2003), an Assertive Community Treatment Technical Assistance Center, and information from the NAMI Policy Research Institute. In 1994, Laurie Flynn, the Executive Director of NAMI charged that "few managed care organizations recognize and provide reimbursement for the full array of services required to maintain seriously mentally ill individuals in the community" (Flynn 1994: 206). In a 1997 study of nine managed behavioral health care companies, NAMI found that managed care is failing to bring the best clinical practices to those with severe mental illnesses (NAMI 1997). The primary problem concerned restrictions to care, especially needed hospitalizations. The NAMI study also found that managed care firms neglected critical community support services, including housing and rehabilitation.[3] In 1998 NAMI surveyed consumer and family experiences with managed care and found that 55 percent did not know how to file an appeal with a managed care company, 41 percent reported an inability to see a doctor, 34 percent had problems getting medication, and 33 percent had problems getting crisis services (NAMI 2003).

In terms of recent activities, NAMI supports passage of the Patients' Bill of Rights (S 283). They also support legislation to allow states to use their Medicaid dollars for Programs for Assertive Community Treatment (PACT). This would increase funding for community-based mental health services for individuals with severe, persistent mental illnesses. PACT is cited as an evidence-based program (and there is good research evidence that PACT does work) and NAMI advocates replication of this program. Supporting PACT is a good way to influence managed care systems to preserve the central principals of community based care. NAMI is also challenging recent Medicaid restrictions on prescription drugs.

Another advocacy group active in the mental health policy arena is the National Mental Health Association. Like NAMI, the NMHA has state affiliates who advocate on the local level while the national organization advocates at the federal level and provides technical assistance to its affiliates. The NMHA has focused most of its efforts on mental health parity. In 1996 the Mental Health Parity Act (P.L. 1040204) was passed. As of 2003, thirty-three states have some form of mental health parity law, although many only cover a small number of mental illnesses. NAMI supports extension of parity to all disorders covered by the DSM-IV. The idea behind parity is to equalize physical and mental health by eliminating the more common restrictions placed on mental health benefits (such as different annual reimbursement levels and lifetime caps). While parity laws are having some effect on mental health benefits (Buck et al. 1999), parity legislation only applies to those employers who offer some kind of mental health benefit and does not apply to firms with fewer than fifty employees or to those firms whose plan premiums would increase by more than one percent because of mental health parity (Jenson et al. 1998).

Because of these limits to the Parity Act, Congress considered new legislation in 2002 (the Mental Health Equitable Treatment Act). This legislation failed to pass, and the existing parity law remains in effect for another year. However, the bill has been reintroduced (as the Paul Wellstone Mental Health Parity Act) and requires full parity for all mental health conditions listed in the DSM. Even if passed, parity is unlikely to increase mental health care benefits because managed care limits services to those considered medically necessary and excludes many services needed by those with more serious mental illnesses (Mechanic and McAlpine 1999). However, NAMI's advocacy for PACT models may well change the way in which medical necessity is defined. More fundamentally, equality of access is not assured with equality of benefits (Burnam and Escarce 1999).

Two other advocacy groups are active in mental health reform: The Bazelon Center for Mental Health Law and the National Council on Disability. The Bazelon Center was established in 1972 and is a nonprofit legal advocacy organization for people with mental disabilities. In addition to the report on states' use of managed care described above, the Bazelon Center has also developed a model law for mental health reform (Bazelon 2001). The Bazelon Center also publishes a number of reports dealing with various aspects of care and support as well as mental health law in their ongoing effort to protect consumer rights. In 1999 they tackled the question of defining medical necessity in managed care systems, and charged that most state contracts granted managed care companies too much discretion in defining medical necessity. A definition of medical necessity has been developed, along with guidelines for service delivery systems (Bazelon Center for Mental Health Law 1999). The Bazelon Center is an excellent resource for both consumers and service providers because they have done the hard work of developing concise standards of care. The National Council on Disability has also published a recent report on mental health services that summarizes the existing knowledge base in terms of services for children, adults, and elderly with mental health problems and provides specific guidelines to improve service delivery (2002). The National Council on Disability promotes recovery, encouraging individuals with mental illness to succeed in the community (ibid.). Their vision calls for fundamental reforms to both existing systems and ways of thinking about individuals with mental disabilities.

There have also been various legislative efforts on the behalf of providers and clients. Any-willing-provider (AWP) laws force managed care firms to accept all qualified providers who agree to a company's terms. These laws have the potential to curb managed care's propensity to limit networks to preferred providers. While twenty-four states had such laws in 1996, the majority were passed before 1994. In 1995, seventy-nine AWP laws were considered but only three passed (Tuttle and Woods 1997), reflecting the lobbying power of the managed care industry. In response, provider groups have turned to right-to-know (forcing managed care companies to state why a provider is dropped from a plan) and point-of-service measures (ibid.). Providers and consumers are also seeking to have practice guidelines made public; they rightfully view the managed care company's control over such standards as a source of great power over treatment decisions and reimbursement. Some states have turned to the use of quality report cards (Carpinello et al. 1998) and a series of legislative efforts have sought to define and protect patient's rights.

These various advocacy efforts arose in response to managed care's threat to community-based care. They provide evidence of the countervailing power of various professional and community groups who seek to oppose managed care companies' clinical decisions. The question remains whether these attempts to protect the quality of care will be able to counter the forces behind the commodification of care.

NOTES

1. My information on the reform movement in North Carolina is a result of my own role as a board member of the Mecklenburg Mental Health Authority, and

from information made available to mental health services researchers at a series of seminars and presentations.

2. It is interesting that the state did not make any provision for an evaluation of the system reform; in fact, the state division has no research funding at all.

3. Yet NAMI has also been instrumental in institutionalizing a biological approach to mental illness, which has had the paradoxical effect under managed care of limiting the very types of social supports needed by those with serious mental illnesses.

9 Market-Based Care?
Prospects for the Future

There is a general feeling of helplessness and depression related to being in fear, and as far as I'm concerned, if people don't have their health, they don't have anything. And there is a real sense of sadness and helplessness. (MSW case manager in nonprofit agency)

I am reminded of a phrase frequently repeated by both providers and clients when I asked them about the future of mental health care: "When you get to the end of your rope, tie a knot and hang on." Individuals with mental illness are often at the end of their ropes, and it is their therapist or case manager who helps them tie that knot by providing needed emotional support. Yet the ability of providers to develop and maintain an intense emotional relationship with clients has been thwarted by wider institutional pressures that constrain their ability to meet their client's needs. When providers are prevented from doing the emotional labor they feel is necessary for the client's well-being and when they are not allowed to act on the basis of their professionally based treatment ideology (which specifies the appropriate feeling rules for the completion of emotional labor), they are likely to experience burnout. The critical organizational conditions of work that contribute to burnout are those which affect the providers' identity, self-image, and sense of personal accomplishment.

Managed care is the most recent institutional demand, and it mandates that treatment meet the wider goal of cost containment and efficacy. Under managed care, the treatment decisions and work practices of providers are subject to third-party review and increasingly, are standardized. The qualitative data analyzed in the previous chapters demonstrate that many clinicians now find themselves at the end of that proverbial rope, and are struggling to tie a knot and hang on in the face of the gale force winds of managed care. This chapter examines providers' beliefs and expectations about the future more closely. Before proceeding to a consideration of the future, I will summarize the major conclusions and insights of the previous chapters.

SUMMARY OF KEY POINTS

In Chapter 2, I examined conflicting beliefs about the etiology of mental illness and the implications of different etiologies for treatment and care. I described three different approaches to mental illness: the psychosocial, the biomedical, and labeling or social reaction theory, and showed that shifting preferences for care reflect wider institutional beliefs, expectations, and priorities (i.e., institutional demands or rational myths) about mental health and treatment. At a broad level of generalization, there has been a shift away from institutional, custodial care to community-based care with a concomitant emphasis upon client normalization (fitting into one's community and meeting social expectations) and client empowerment (giving the client greater autonomy and self-determination and allowing the client to not fit in). Normalization and empowerment have contradictory implications for treatment. Normalization contributes to the social control functions of labeling by creating an expectation that the individual will conform to social norms, while empowerment explicitly rejects professional interventions and conformity to the status quo. Recovery is a more recent model that combines both normalization and empowerment and advocates the development of collaborative relationships between providers and consumers (Jacobson and Greenley 2001).

The majority of providers whom I interviewed felt that mental illness could be best understood and treated from a broad biopsychosocial perspective that views mental illness as having biological, psychological, and sociological components. Providers in private practice were least likely to emphasize the biological aspects of mental illness and placed greater emphasis upon psychological factors. Providers in private practice were also more likely to work with clients with acute types of mental illnesses or problems and to emphasize therapy. Providers working with clients with more severe mental illnesses were more likely to be in the public sector. These providers were case managers rather than therapists and their role was to coordinate the various community supports needed by their clients. Case managers are more likely to view treatment in terms of psychosocial rehabilitation although the majority felt that medication played an important role in providing "baseline" treatment. In fact, most case managers believed that clients needed to become stabilized on medication before psychosocial rehabilitation would be effective. However, given persistent resource constraints on the availability of effective psychosocial rehabilitation and needed community support, case managers also felt frustrated by what they perceived to be an over-reliance on medication as the primary form of treatment. I suggested that providers were frustrated by the limitations case management placed upon their emotional labor, and by the prevailing models of community-based care that emphasized the coordination of social services rather than the development of a therapeutic relationship with clients. In short, case management has the potential to curtail the emotional labor of mental health professionals who become managers, rather than providers, of care. Consequently, these workers are likely to experience psychological burnout, and indeed, burnout was the prevalent concern in both the academic literature and among mental health professionals during the 1980s and early 1990s, when community-based care was in its ascendancy.

In Chapter 3, I examined the treatment ideologies of providers. Treatment ideologies encompass the feeling rules that direct the emotional labor of providers, and specify the appropriate role of the provider as well the goal of treatment. Treatment ideologies are central to providers' views of themselves and their work identities. At the same time, treatment ideologies are collective in nature (they are properties of groups), and are central features of the culture as well as the formal structure of the organizations in which they are enacted. Treatment ideologies also exist outside of the organization, especially in the form of professionally based normative expectations about mental health care, for example, the preference for community-based care. Treatment ideologies are therefore likely to be an important source of professional conflict, as different groups of providers (whether linked by education or work role), seek to see a given treatment ideology implemented within the organization. Different professional orientations are one potential source of conflict between treatment ideologies, ambiguous institutional demands are another, and conflict between the ideal proscriptions (fundamental aspects of the treatment ideology) and realistic goals of treatment (operative aspects) are a third. Mediatory myths play an important role in helping providers resolve ideological contradictions; providers were able to resolve contradictions between medication and psychosocial therapy by believing that medication compliance was a prerequisite for effective treatment.

A typology of treatment ideologies was also presented in Chapter 3. The typology is based upon two axes: (1) the appropriate role of the provider and (2) the appropriate goal of treatment. In examining the prevalence of the six theoretical treatment ideologies among providers working in two mental health care programs, I found the most widely held treatment ideology (adhered to by a little over one-third of the providers) emphasized normalization, the second was caretaking, and the third was reparenting. All three ideologies are consistent with the wider institutional framework of biopsychosocial rehabilitation, and emphasize the adjustment of the client as the primary goal of treatment (caretaking and reparenting) or autonomy (normalization), and view the role of the provider as primarily supportive (caretaking and normalization) or facilitative (reparenting). Relatively few providers adhered to more custodial treatment ideologies, nor did many adhere to an ideology organized around client empowerment (which also exists within the wider framework of community-based care).

Debates over the future of community mental health care systems will be determined in part by the providers' support for alternative ideologies of care. As Hasenfeld (1992: 13–14) has noted, evaluations about the effectiveness of services involve "moral choices that are embedded in the practice ideologies" of providers. However, it is important to keep in mind that the typology of treatment ideologies developed in Chapter 3 is not meant to portray a closed system; rather, it is historically framed by the institutional expectations and rational myths about mental illness and treatment prevalent during the 1980s and 1990s, when community-based care was organized around a biopsychosocial paradigm. New treatment ideologies will emerge with new institutional demands and professionals groups.

Managed care is a major institutional demand that has the result of increasing the degree of bureaucratic control over clinical work. In Chapter 4, I argue that managed care should not be understood in terms of the traditional bureaucratic model in which organizational structures produce efficient outcomes; instead, managed care exemplifies the commodity model (Meyer 1990) in which organizational structures are the products of wider institutional demands for efficiency. The technocratic rationality of the commodity model is driven the by specific goal of cost-containment (in the public sector) or the accumulation of profit (in the private sector).

Financial imperatives have been the primary institutional force driving the delivery of mental health since the mid 1980s. However, the institutional demand for cost-containment (which itself results in a focus upon efficiency) is fundamentally in conflict with professionally based logics of mental health care. Community-based care and psychosocial rehabilitation emphasize community integration rather than the alleviation of specific symptoms, long-term care as opposed to short-term interventions, and the development of the adaptive capacities of the clients rather than merely functional improvement. Consequently, providers must negotiate between contradictory institutional demands in their work practices, and these contradictions are experienced as a series of ethical dilemmas. Providers also felt that mechanisms for the review of treatment decisions by managed care entities limited their autonomy, and had the potential to reduce the quality of care received by clients.

In Chapter 5, I explored the organizations within which providers carry out their work, and examined the conflict between bureaucratic and professional authority, as well as the consequences of managed care for working conditions and service offerings in public mental health care organizations. There was evidence in the qualitative data of jurisdictional disputes, especially within treatment teams where providers had to collaborate to make decisions about client care. These conflicts in part reflected different treatment ideologies, and were not problematic where differences of opinion were treated with respect. Organizational context was critical in allowing for the resolution of professional conflict.

In Chapter 5, I described in detail one public sector approach to managed care, which has sought to preserve the principles of community-based care. CARE seeks to increase access to mental health services to the entire community as well as to preserve the comprehensive, continuous and integrated system of services needed by those with severe mental illness. Through an extensive system of contracts with private agencies, CARE is also on its way to eliminating the two-tiered system of care. Despite a great deal of professional involvement, and concern to maintain a high quality system of care to clients with severe mental illness, empirical evidence demonstrates that providers were very dissatisfied with managed care, and felt that it undermined the care for clients with long-term care needs. There was less emphasis on the provision of the services and supports necessary for community stability (as measured by the Community Program Philosophy Scale). Furthermore, the work environment was less supportive because of lower levels of job involvement, reduced role clarity, and lower levels of group cohesion under managed care. Providers also reported less satisfaction with work and lower levels of autonomy, as well as higher levels of burnout.

The organization in which providers work is essential to understanding burnout, but poor organizational working conditions do not directly result in burnout. Emotional labor is also a crucial factor. It requires an investment of self in the treatment role in order to maintain a relationship with one's client. In Chapter 6, I argued that burnout results when the organization prevents providers from performing the kind of emotional labor they deem necessary for effective care of clients. Rather than controlling the emotional labor of providers, organizational constraints on treatment practices make it difficult for the provider to have the feelings and act in the way in which they have been trained to do. The critical organizational conditions of work that contribute to burnout are those which affect one's work identity and sense of personal accomplishment. I suggested that when managed care reduces the professional prerogative of providers burnout is exacerbated. Managed care imposes an additional layer of bureaucracy on providers already overwhelmed by paperwork, and constrains their emotional labor by dictating what type of treatment will be made available.

In Chapter 7, I examined the effect of managed care on providers' experience of burnout. The comments of providers showed that managed care contributed to increased levels of burnout. Providers in private practice were almost universally critical of managed care, and described the ways in which utilization review had changed treatment practices and limited the types and availability of services to clients with private, employer-based insurance. Providers in the public sector also felt that managed care had changed their work, and expressed a great deal of frustration and resentment about the constraints on the care available to their clients. Disagreement with organizational priorities which placed cost-containment goals above client care was a significant source of burnout, as was a lack of professional control and the sense that one's work was not meaningful. While burnout is a type of alienation from one's work and identity, further commodification of care may entail a greater dehumanization of mental health care.

Chapter 8 focused on recent institutional forces that have had an impact on mental health care services. I first examined efforts to integrate professional based logics of care with the institutional logic of cost-containment and commodification. Standards for quality care may be the vehicle by which this integration can be achieved, and I described current efforts to develop and implement quality measures of performance. I also looked at the impact of another institutional force: legislation, focusing on the situation in North Carolina mandating the privatization of public sector mental health. Other critical pieces of legislation that will influence mental health services include the Patient Bill of Rights, the Mental Health Parity Act, and legislation allowing states to use Medicaid dollars for eviden-based community services. The large number of groups advocating for consumers and for systems of care that allow for their recovery are evidence of countervailing power. They offer hope that quality care will not be sacrificed in the name of cost-containment.

One limitation to my study has been that much of the data about the effects of managed care comes from one agency (CARE) and from a small number of providers in private practice in one region of the country. As has been noted, there is tremendous variability in mental health systems and the degree of managed care penetration. There is also tremendous variability in the experiences and practices of mental health care providers. Consequently, I have utilized data available in the literature from private practice clinicians to augment my own findings, as well as a case study of a private, nonprofit managed care organization in another state. CARE is an important case in its own right (as the first public sector agency to received national certification by the National Committee for Quality Assurance as a Managed Behavioral Health Organization). This organization is both substantively as well as theoretically significant (Berg 1990; Ragin 1999) and my study leads to a deeper understanding of how managed mental health care works. The data I have collected from CARE over time allowed me to examine the institutional logics that drive changes in the provision of services, and to consider if professional logics can be preserved. Furthermore, the organization of care and working conditions as well as experience of burnout at CARE prior to managed care are similar to those of nineteen mental health programs in Wisconsin. I use in-depth data from another Wisconsin program (SUPPORT) in the development of my arguments. However, further research on the effect of managed care on mental health organizations and care work is clearly needed.

THE FUTURE OF MENTAL HEALTH CARE WORK

My interviews with providers generally ended with questions about the future of mental health care; I would ask "Where do you think you will be in ten years," and, "Where do you think mental health care will be in ten years?" The responses in recent years have been overwhelming negative, and contrast sharply with the more positive responses given in the early 1990s when the community-based care promised to offer integrated community-support programs that could indeed coordinate the diverse services needed by clients with long-term mental health care problems.

As noted in the previous chapter, providers in private practice were extremely cynical about the future. Almost 25 percent of providers who completed the questionnaire stated flatly they would retire, and another 25 percent said they were looking for alternative ways to make a living. These responses were blunt and matter-of-fact, as typified by the following MSW. "I have always said before I do straight managed care, I would sell real estate." Regrettably, two of the eleven providers I interviewed in 1997 had indeed left private practice by the following year, both with deep sorrow and regret. Some providers felt there would still be a "market for the self paying patient," and they would be able to serve those clients. However, the majority did not feel they could continue to make a living under managed care and they were actively seeking career alternatives.

In terms of specific changes, providers in private practice believed that there would be more emphasis placed upon accountability and further specialization. They anticipated that the role of psychiatrists would be limited to prescribing medication, and that nurses would eventually fill this role at a cheaper price. Psychologists, especially those who practiced psychotherapy, were also in jeopardy. Overall, they predicted further deprofessionalization of mental health care, as higher priced PhDs and physicians will be replaced by MSWs and nurses. As described in the previous chapters, most providers in private practice felt they had to join a group in order to survive. They anticipated that treatment sessions would become even more narrowly focused around specific questions to the point that providers would become "Dear Abbys [who give] an answer in a thirty-second soundbite."

Three providers held more positive views of the future. They felt that the trend toward managed care would reverse itself; one psychologist felt the "curtailment of care will continue until a massive lawsuit draws attention to the problem." Providers hoped that managed care would become more regulated. One MSW provider felt capitation would actually be beneficial, because there would no longer be "intrusive, case-by-case, utilization review." This was certainly the experience of the Venture non-profit agency that did utilize capitation. However, the MSW provider continued with the following observation:

> It's hard to see how managed care can make the system work better. If the pot of money is such that you can do whatever you need to with a patient, that would be different; but its such a bureaucratic mess . . . managed care will just add another layer of bureaucracy.

In fact, providers at Venture did complain about the increased paperwork of managed care, as well as increased levels of bureaucracy.

Providers in the public sector are more used to bureaucracy, but providers at CARE also felt the amount of paperwork and bureaucratic control of managed care was excessive. While many of the providers at CARE felt that managed care did have the potential to increase efficiency and agreed that too many clients had become dependent on the system to meet needs that might be better met by other groups in the community, they echoed the concerns raised by providers in private practice about the quality of care and the ability of managed care to meet the long-term needs of their clients. Most found that they were serving a larger client population with fewer resources, and had less time to spend with each client.

In their descriptions of the future none of the providers felt that changes in managed care would lead to greater service integration or more effective treatment. Although providers felt that a greater degree of accountability was probably good, they did not necessarily believe that accountability in and of itself would lead to better care. Certainly the mechanisms to ensure accountability (third-party review, authorization, and standardization of treatment practices) decrease the autonomy of the providers, and limit their ability to provide care or to maintain a relationship with their clients. Third-party review undermines the therapeutic relationship by introducing distrust of the clinician, and places constraints on the emotional labor of clinicians. Under these conditions it is anticipated that providers will have lower levels of job satisfaction, and higher levels of burnout, which will have a detrimental affect on the quality of client care. Furthermore, with deprofessionalization and the lowering of fees, it will be harder to retain good providers. As one mental health provider noted, "You are knocked down with a sledgehammer, and then told to provide services."

RECOMMENDATIONS AND IMPLICATIONS

What can providers do to prevent burnout, and to counter those aspects of managed care that could result in poorer quality care? In the private sector the movement toward group practices may in fact produce an important countervailing power. First, providers will have the support of peers and colleagues who can help them deal with the frustrations of third-party reviews as well the sense of hopelessness associated with burnout. Second, group organizations can lead to organized resistance; it is much easier for providers to argue with a utilization reviewer if they have the weight of other professional opinions behind them. Just as treatment teams helped providers in the public sector alleviate burnout and gave them needed emotional support, group practices both alleviate burnout and also reinforce professional prerogative. As one MSW provider in private practice argued:

> Group practice—it's the only way to partner with managed care, to have a voice and to be heard. Change won't happen from individuals, but from groups of people.

A critical factor in the ability of diverse professional groups to unite against the technocratic rationality of managed care will be their ability to put aside long-standing disputes and to work together. MSW providers and nurses will be critical to this process; at present they have the most to gain by managed care because their roles will expand. Furthermore, nurses and social workers are using their professional associations to develop and impose ethical standards for care. Yet in the long run they will face the same threats to their professional status as psychologists and psychiatrists now do. It is in everyone's interest to agree that while there are different approaches to the treatment of mental illness, an integrated approach goes furthest to assure that clients have good quality of life. Consumer groups and other advocates must also work with providers to raise awareness of the larger social costs of inadequate mental health care (i.e., caregiver burden, lowered productivity, higher medical costs, costly inpatient care, strains on other parts of the social service system) and to force managed care companies to take these broader costs into account when evaluating treatment effectiveness.

A force more insidious than managed care is managed competition, which results from providers' competing for contracts. Light (2001) argues that managed competition undermines public health. In private practice, managed competition takes place when providers compete to get on panels. Managed care corporations utilize those providers whose fees are the lowest, and who do not seek treatment beyond the limits imposed by insurance plans. Consequently, there is a strong disincentive for providers to work with clients with long-term or in-depth needs. There is potential that the quality of care will decline as "good" therapists are able to either carve out a niche with private-pay clients, or else opt out of mental health altogether.

Managed competition is also a factor in the public sector. Increasingly, providers are competing for public sector contracts for Medicaid. CARE has developed a model where internal providers (those employed by CARE) are outsourced and have to compete with providers in the private sector for a contract to provide services or treatment. This model has now been mandated for the entire state of North Carolina. While managed competition will surely result in care that is more cost effective and perhaps even "better" in terms of quality, competition will further divide mental health care professionals and leave them with little organizational clout to battle those managed care entities whose primary concern is "to manage the dollars rather than the care." It is critical for governmental agencies who purchase services to set high standards for quality care (Lehman 1999).

As noted by Schlesinger and Gray (1999: 436) professional norms have not played a major role in the diffusion of managed care. While the broader shift toward technical rationality conflicts with professionally based norms, providers have exhibited deep ambivalence about managed care. When providers play a role in developing, implementing, and evaluating managed care guidelines and clinical standards they preserve a degree of professional prerogative. Rather than accepting the growing constraints on their work, providers must demand input into the bureaucratic structures designed to manage care and fight for the services needed by those clients most likely to suffer under managed care (i.e., those with chronic conditions and long-term care needs). For example, providers should not allow utilization review to become a distinct specialty that is performed by individuals with little direct contact with clients; instead they should demand representation and the right to set the standards by which treatment decisions are evaluated. Providers should also ask that clients be allowed a voice in those decisions that affect treatment, a position that is consistent with a broader emphasis upon empowerment.

Utilization review should be decentralized, not deprofessionalized. Centralization begets further bureaucracy, and raises the administrative costs of care. Decentralization of external review will maximize efficiencies. Furthermore, as a long tradition of organizational research has repeatedly demonstrated (Scott 1992), bureaucratic control is incompatible with high levels of technical or environmental uncertainty, and both conditions characterize mental health care. When environmental expectations are ambiguous, contradictory and/or uncertain, and treatment technologies highly variable in their effectiveness (as is typical of mental health care), a multitude of exceptions to the standardized procedures arise, as do solutions characteristic of formalized systems of control. Problems are consequently referred upward, the system becomes overwhelmed, and yet another new organizational form must be created to solve the new problems (Galbraith 1973). For example, in addition to utilization review committees, CARE created a separate committee to handle appeals. Hierarchical structures also lead to increased role strains and conflict (Guy 1985) between those with different degrees of power as well as between different professional and occupational work groups. Flatter organizational hierarchies and participatory decision making not only have the potential to decrease burnout and increase job satisfaction, but they will also promote the development of creative, interdisciplinary solutions to mental health problems and client care.

Providers are currently accepting the constraints imposed by managed care because they have developed a mediatory myth that helps them to reconcile the contradictions between the technocratic rationality of managed care and their own professionally based logics of care. That is, providers believe that increased accountability leads to better care for more clients. And this "myth" is valid; but providers must ask hard questions about the system designed to provide for that accountability: must accountability be measured by those whose primary concern is with cost-containment, rather than client care? Professional associations need to develop standards by which care is measured, and the standards of different professional groups must respect the diversity of treatment approaches characteristic of mental health care. Mental health care is based on emotional labor, which develops and maintains a relationship between a provider and a client. Even prescribing and administering medication involves emotional labor. Treatment protocols need to be organized around those principles that allow providers to do their emotional labor in the manner which best serves their clients; that is, according to their professional norms.

Herron (1997) argues that we need to attack managed care head-on by demonstrating that there is no cost crisis in outpatient psychotherapy and that more mental health care is *better* health care. The broader social benefits of enhanced mental health is an area that has not received much research attention; instead researchers emphasizing accountability have set the agenda by focusing on the measurement and prediction of narrowly defined client-level outcomes. In short, both providers and researchers need to challenge the institutional logic of technical rationality and insist that mental health care be measured by a wider social ethic than that of cost-containment. As Mechanic (1999: xii) has eloquently argued:

> Managed care is simply a framework. What takes place in this framework will continue to be affected by our economic and social philosophies and values and by our conceptions about the nature of mental health and illness.

Mental health, as well as physical health, is a social good, and we need to ask ourselves if health care systems should be organized around professionally based ethical standards of care or upon principles of cost-containment and technical rationality. We must also determine who sets the standards by which accountability is being assessed, and what view of mental health is used to define and evaluate outcomes. Providers must address these questions, and work collectively with consumer groups and advocates to design delivery systems that contain the social costs of mental illness.

References

Abbott, Andrew. 1988. *The System of Professions*. Chicago: University of Chicago Press.
————. 1992. "Professional Work." Pp. 145–162 in *Human Services as Complex Organizations*, edited by Y. Hasenfeld. Newbury Park: Sage.
Abravanel, Henry. 1983. "Mediatory Myths in the Service of Organizational Ideology." Pp. 273–293 in *Organizational Symbolism*, edited by L. Pondy, P. J. Frost, G. Morgan, and T. Dandridge. Greenwich, CT: JAI Press.
Aches, Joan. 1991. "Social Structure, Burnout, and Job Satisfaction." *Social Work* 36: 202–206.
Aday, Lu Ann, Charles E. Begley, David R. Lairson and Carl H. Slater. 1993. *Evaluating the Medical Care System*. Ann Arbor: Health Administration Press.
Ahmed, Paul I., and Stanley C. Plog (eds.). 1976. *State Mental Hospitals: What Happens When They Close?* New York: Plenum Medical Book Co.
Aiken, Linda H., and Douglas M. Sloan. 1997. "Effects of Specialization and Client Differentiation on the Status of Nurses: The Case of Aids." *Journal of Health and Social Behavior* 38: 203–222.
Alexander, Jeffrey A., and Terry L. Amburgey. 1987. "The Dynamics of Change in the American Hospital Industry: Transformation or Selection." *Medical Care Review* 44: 279–321.
Alexander, Jeffrey A., and Thomas A. D'Aunno. 1990. "Transformation of Institutional Environments: Perspectives on the Corporatization of U.S. Health Care." Pp. 53–85 in *Innovations in Health Care Delivery*, edited by Stephen S. Mick et al. San Francisco: Jossey-Bass.
Alperin, Richard M., and David G. Phillips (editors). 1997. *The Impact of Managed Care on the Practice of Psychotherapy*. New York: Brunner/Mazel Publishers.
American Psychiatric Association. 1994. *Diagnostic and Statistical Manual of Mental Disorders (Fourth Edition) (DSM-IV)*. Washington, DC.
Anderlik, Mary R. 2001. *The Ethics of Managed Care: A Pragmatic Approach*. Bloomington, IN: Indiana University Press.
Anderson, James G. 1992. "The Deprofessionalization of American Medicine." *Current Research in Occupations and Professions* 7: 241–256.
Anderton, Joan M., Helen Elfert, and Magdalene Lai. 1989. "Ideology in the Clinical Context: Chronic Illness, Ethnicity, and the Discourse of Normalization." *Sociology of Health and Illness* 11: 253–278.

Andresky, Lisa M. 1996. "Burnout and Job Dissatisfaction: An Examination of the Role Played by Job Control, Personal and Organizational Characteristics." MA Thesis, University of North Carolina at Charlotte.

Anspach, Renne. 1991. "Everyday Methods for Assessing Organizational Effectiveness." *Social Problems* 38: 1–19.

Ashforth, Blake E., and Ronald H. Humphrey. 1993. "Emotional Labor in Service Roles: The Influence of Identity." *Academy of Management Review* 18: 88–115.

Atwood, Nancy. 1982. "Professional Prejudice and the Psychotic Client." *Social Work* 27: 172–177.

Austad, Carol S., and Michael F. Hoyt. 1992. "The Managed Care Movement and the Future of Psychotherapy." *Psychotherapy* 19: 109–118.

Aviram, Uri. 1990. "Community Care of the Seriously Mentally Ill." *Community Mental Health Journal* 26: 69–88.

Bacharach, S., P. Bamberg, and S. Conley. 1990. "Work Processes, Role Conflict, and Role Overload." *Sociology of Work and Occupations* 17: 199–28.

Bachrach, Lenore L. 1996. "Patients' Quality of Life: A Continuing Concern in the Literature." *Psychiatric Services* 47: 1305–6.

Backlar, Patricia. 1996. "Managed Mental Health Care: Conflicts of Interest in the Provider/Client Relationship." *Community Mental Health Journal* 32: 101–106.

Barley, Stephen R., and Deborah B. Knight. 1992. "Toward a Cultural Theory of Stress Complaints." *Research in Organizational Behavior* 14: 1–48.

Baszanger, Isabelle. 1985. "Professional Socialization as Social Control: From Medical Students to General Practitioners." *Social Science and Medicine* 20: 133–143.

Baum, Joel and Christine Oliver. 1991. "Institutional Linkages and Organizational Mortality." *Administrative Science Quarterly* 36: 187–218.

Bayley, Michael. 1991. "Normalization or 'Social Role' Valorization: An Adequate Philosophy?" Pp. 87–99 in *Mental Handicap: Social Sciences Perspectives,* edited by S. Baldwin and J. Hattersley. New York: Routledge.

Bazelon Center for Mental Health Law. 1995. "Managing Managed Care for Publicly Financed Mental Health Services." Washington, DC. See http://www.bazelon.org.

———. "Defining Medically Necessary' Services to Protect Plan Members. Washington, DC. See http://www.bazelon.org.

———. 2000. "Effective Public Management of Mental Health Care: Views from States on Medicaid Reforms That Enhance Service System Integration and Accountability." Washington, DC. See http://www.bazelon.org.

———. 2001a. "Disintegrating Systems: The State of State's Public Mental Health Systems." Washington, DC. See http://www.bazelon.org.

———. 2001b. "A New Version of Public Mental Health: A Model Law to Provide a Right to Mental Health Services and Supports." Washington, DC. See http://www.bazelon.org.

Becker, Howard S., Blanche Geer, Everett C. Hughes, and Anselm L. Strauss. 1961. *Boys in White: The Student Culture in Medical School.* Chicago: University of Chicago Press.

Beigel, Allan, Kenneth Minkoff, and Miles Shore. 1997. "Research: System, Program and Clinician Level Measures." Pp. 309–320 in *Managed Mental Health Care in the Public Sector,* edited by K. Minkoff and D. Pollack. The Netherlands: Harwood Academic Publishers.

Ben-Dror, Raphael. 1994. "Employee Turnover in Community Mental Health Organizations: A Developmental Stages Model." *Community Mental Health Journal* 30: 243–257.

Benner, Patricia. 1984. *From Novice to Expert: Excellence and Power in Clinical Nursing Practice*. Menlo Park, CA: Addison-Wesley.

Bensman, Joseph and Robert Lilienfeld. 1991. *Craft and Consciousness: Occupational Technique and the Development of World Images*, 2e. New York: Aldine de Gruyter.

Berg, David. 1990. "A Case in Print." *The Journal of Applied Behavioral Science* 26: 67–70.

Berger, Peter and Thomas Luckman. 1967. *The Social Construction of Reality*. New York: Anchor Books.

———, Bridgette Berger, and Hansfried Kellner. 1973. *The Homeless Mind*. New York: Random House.

Bergman, Jorg R. 1992. "Veiled Morality: Notes on Discretion in Psychiatry." Pp. 137–162 in *Talk at Work: Interaction in Institutional Settings*, edited by P. Drew and J. Heritage. Cambridge: Cambridge University Press.

Berkman, Barbara, E. Bonander, I. Ruthchick, P. Silverman, B. Kemler, L. Marcus, M-J. Isacson-Rubiner. 1990. "Social Work in Health Care: Directions in Practice." *Social Science and Medicine* 31: 19–26.

Birne-Stone, Susan, Adrienne Cypres, and Steven Winderbaum. 1997. "Case-Management and Review Strategies." Pp. 51–56 in *The Impact of Managed Care on the Practice of Psychotherapy*, edited by R. M. Alperin and D. G. Phillips 1997. New York: Brunner/Mazel Publishers.

Blue Ribbon Commission. 1997. *The Wisconsin Blue Ribbon Commission on Mental Health: Final Report*. Submitted to Tommy G. Thompson, Governor of Wisconsin.

Bockoven, J. Sanbourne. 1972. *Moral Treatment in Community Mental Health*. New York: Springer.

Bosk, Charles L. 1979. *Forgive and Remember: Managing Medical Failure*. Chicago: University of Chicago Press.

Boyle, P. J., and D. Callahan. 1995. "Managed Care in Mental Health: The Ethical Issues." *Health Affairs* 14: 7–23.

Brekke, J. S., and M. A. Test. 1992. "A Model for Measuring and Implementation of Community Support Programs: Results From Three Sites." *Community Mental Health Journal* 28: 227–247.

Brotheridge, Celeste and Alicia Grady. 2002. "Emotional Labor and Burnout: Comparing Two Perspectives of 'People Work.'" *Journal of Vocational Behavior*, 60: 17–39.

Broman, Clifford, William S. Hoffman, and V. Lee Hamilton. 1994. Impact of Mental Health Services Use on Subsequent Mental Health of Autoworkers. *Journal of Health and Social Behavior* 35: 80–95.

Brown, P., and E. Cooksey. 1989. "Mental Health Monopoly: Corporate Trends in Mental Health Services." *Social Science and Medicine* 28: 1129–1139.

Buck, Jeffrey A., Judith L. Teich, Beth Umland, and Mitchell Stein. 1999. "Behavioral Health Benefits in Employer Sponsored Health Plans 1997." *Health Affairs* 18: 67–78.

———, and Beth Umland. 1997. "Covering Mental Health and Substance Abuse Services." *Health Affairs* 16: 120–126.

Bulen, Hether F., Rebecca J. Erickson, and Amy S. Wharton. 1997. "Doing for Others on the Job: The Affective Requirements of Service Work, Gender, and Emotional Well Being." *Social Problems* 44: 235–256.

Burfoot, Jean. 1994. "Outlaw Emotions and the Sensual Dynamics of Compassion." Presented at the 1994 *American Sociological Association Meetings*, Los Angeles.

Burke, Ronald and Ester Greenglass. 1995. "A Longitudinal Examination of the Cherniss Model of Psychological Burnout." *Social Science and Medicine* 40: 1357–1363.

———. 1999. "A Longitudinal Examination of Psychological Burnout in Teachers." *Human Relations* 48: 187–202.

Burnam, M. Audrey and Jose J. Escarce. 1998. "Equity in Managed Care for Mental Disorders." *Health Affairs* 18: 22–31.

Callahan, Daniel. 1994. "Setting Mental Health Priorities: Problems and Possibilities." *The Millibank Quarterly* 72: 451–470.

Cameron, Kim S., and Whetton, David A. (eds.). 1983. *Organizational Effectiveness: A Comparison of Multiple Models.* New York: Academic Press.

Campbell, S. M., and M. O. Roland, and S. A. Buetow. 2000. "Defining Quality of Care." *Social Science and Medicine* 51: 1611–1625.

Caplan, Paula J. 1995. *They Say You're Crazy: How the World's Most Powerful Psychiatrists Decide Who's Normal.* Reading, MA: Addison-Wesley.

Carney, J., R. Donavan, M. Yurdin, R. Starr, A. Pernell-Arnold, and E. M. Bromberg. 1993. "Incidence of Burnout among NYC Intensive Case Managers." *Psychosocial Rehabilitation Journal* 16: 26–38.

Carpinello, Sharon, Chip J. Felton, Elizabeth A. Peace, Mary DeMasis, and Sheila Donahue. 1998. "Designing a System for Managing the Performance of Mental Health Managed Care: An Example from New York State's Prepaid Mental Health Plan." *The Journal of Behavioral Health Services and Research* 25: 269–278.

Center for Quality Assesment and Improvement in Mental Health. 2003. "National Inventory of Mental Health Quality Measures. See http://www.cqaimh.org.

Chamberlain, Judi. 1979. *On Our Own: Patient-Controlled Alternatives to Mental Health Systems.* New York: Hawthorn.

Chambliss, Daniel. 1996. *Beyond Caring: Hospitals, Nurses, and the Social Organization of Ethics.* Chicago: University of Chicago Press.

Chandler, Susan M. 1990. *Competing Realities: The Contested Terrain of Mental Health Advocacy.* New York: Praeger.

Cherniss, Cary. 1980. *Staff Burnout: Job Stress in the Human Services.* Beverly Hills, CA: Sage.

Clark, R. E., R. A. Dorwart, and S. S. Epstein. 1994. "Managing Competition in Public and Private Mental Health Agencies: Implications for Services and Policy." *The Milibank Quarterly* 72: 653–678.

Cicourel, Aaron V. 1968. *Method and Measurement in Sociology.* New York: The Free Press.

Cohen, M. and D. Wagner. 1982. "Social Work Professionalism: Reality and Illusion." Pp. 141–162 in *Professionals as Workers: Mental Labor in Advanced Capitalism,* edited by C. Derber. Boston: CK Hall and Co.

Conrad, Peter. 1990. "Qualitative Research on Chronic Illness: A Commentary on Method and Conceptual Development." *Social Science and Medicine* 30: 1257–1263.

Cook, Judith and Eric Wright. 1995. "Medical Sociology and the Study of Severe Mental Illnesses: Reflections on Past Accomplishments and Directions for Future Research." *Journal of Health and Social Behavior* Special Issue: 95–114.

Cordes, Cynthia L. and Thomas W. Dougherty. 1993. "A review and integration of research into job burnout." *Academy of Management Review* 18: 621–656.

Coulter, Jeff. 1973. *Approaches to Insanity: A Philosophical and Sociological Study.* New York: John Wiley & Sons.

Croze, Collete. 2000. "Managed Behavioral Healthcare in the Public Sector." *Administration and Policy in Mental Health* 28: 23–36.

Daft, Richard L. and Karl E. Weick. 1984. "Toward a Model of Organizations as Interpretation Systems." *Academy of Managament Review* 9: 284–295.

D'Aunno, Thomas. 1991. "The Effectiveness of Human Service Organizations: A Comparison of Models." Pp. 341–361 in *Human Services as Complex Organizations,* edited by Y. Hasenfeld. Newbury Park, CA: Sage Publications.

———, Robert. I. Sutton, Richard Price. 1991. "Isomorphism and External Support in Conflicting Institutional Environments: A Study of Drug Abuse Treatment Units." *Academy of Management Review* 34: 636–661.

Davies, Celia. 1983. "Professionals in Bureaucracies: The Conflict Thesis Revisited." Pp. 117–194 in *The Sociology of the Professions,* edited by R. Dingwall and P. Lewis. New York: St. Martins Press.

Deitchman, Walter S. 1980. "How Many Case Managers Does It Take to Screw in a Light Bulb?" Open Forum in *Hospital & Community Psychiatry* 31: 788–789.

Devers, Kelly J., Shoshanna Sofaer, and Thomas G. Rundall. 2000. "Introduction to the Special Issue on Qualitative Methods in Health Services Research." *Health Services Research* 34. Part II: 1–6.

Dill, Ann P. 1994. "Institutional Environments and Organizational Responses to AIDS." *Journal of Health and Social Behavior* 35: 349–369.

———. 2001. *Managing to Care: Case Management and Service System Reform.* New York: Aldine de Gruyter.

———, and David Rochefort. 1989. "Coordination, Continuity, and Centralized Control: A Policy Perspective on Service Strategies for the Chronic Mentally Ill." *Journal of Social Issues* 45: 145–159.

DiMaggio, Walter and Walter W. Powell. 1983. "The Iron Cage Revisited: Institutional Isomorphism and Collective Rationality in Organizational Fields." *American Sociological Review* 48: 147–160.

———. 1991. "Introduction." Pp. 1–38 in *The New Institutionalism in Organizational Analysis.* Chicago: University of Chicago Press.

Dingwall, Robert and Philip Lewis. 1983. *The Sociology of the Professions: Lawyers, Doctors and Others.* New York: St. Martins Press.

Dobbin, F. R., L. Edelman, J. W. Meyer, W. R. Scott and A. Swidler. 1988. "The Expansion of Due Process in Organizations." Pp. 147–160 in *Institutional Patterns and Organizations: Culture and Environment,* edited by L. Zucker. Cambridge, MA: Ballenger Publishings.

Doherty, Edmund G., and Josepth Harry. 1976. "Structural Dissensus in a Therapeutic Community." *Journal of Health and Social Behavior* 17: 272–279.

Dottl, Sue L., and James R. Greenley. 1994. "Overview of the Core Data Base of the Mental Health Research Center." MHRC Research Series Paper (No. 42), University of Wisconsin.

Doubt, Keith. 1992. "Mead's Theory of Self and Schizophrenia." *The Social Science Journal* 29: 307–321.

Dowdall, Gerald. 1996. *The Eclipse of the State Mental Hospital: Policy, Stigma and Organization.* Albany, NY: State University of New York Press.

Drolen, Carol S. 1990. "Current Community Mental Health Center Operations: Entrepreneurship or Business as Usual?" *Community Mental Health Journal* 26: 547–558.

Durham, Mary L. 1995. "Can HMOs Manage the Mental Health Benefit?" *Health Affairs* 14: 116–122.

Eaton, William, Christian Ritter, and Diane Brown. 1990. "Psychiatric Epidemiology and Psychiatric Sociology: Influences on the Recognition of Bizarre Behaviors as Social Problems." Pp. 41–68 in *Research in Community Mental Health* (Vol 6), edited by James R. Greenley. Greenwich, CT: JAI Press.

Edelman, Lauren B. 1992. "Legal Ambiguity and Symbolic Structures: Organizational Mediation of Civil Rights Law." *American Journal of Sociology* 97: 1531–1564.

Edwards, Joyce. 1997. "The Impact of Managed Care on the Psychoanalytic Psychotherapeautic Process." Pp. 199–216 in R. M. Alperin and D. G. Phillips. New York: Brunner/Mazel Publishers.

Edwards, Joyce. 1999. "Is Managed Mental Health Treatment Psychotherapy?" *Clinical Social Work Journal* 27: 87–102.

Eisenberg, Leon. 1995. "The Social Construction of the Brain." *American Journal of Psychiatry* 152: 1563–1571.

Engel, George L. 1980. "The Clinical Application of the Biopsychosocial Model." *American Journal of Psychiatry* 137: 525–544.

England, Paula and Nancy Folbre. 1999. "The Costs of Caring." Pp. 39–51 in *Emotional Labor in the Service Economy: Special Issues of the Annals of the American Academy of Political and Social Sciences. Vol 561*, edited by Ronnie J. Steinberg and Deborah M. Figard. Thousand Oaks, CA: Sage.

Erickson, Rebecca J. 1995. "The Importance of Authenticity for Self and Society." *Symbolic Interaction* 18: 117–136.

———, and Amy S. Wharton. 1997. "Inauthenticity and Depression: Assessing the Consequences of Interactive Service Work." *Work and Occupations* 24: 188–213.

———, and Christian Ritter. 2001. "Emotional Labor, Burnout and Inauthenticity: Does Gender Matter?" *Social Psychological Quarterly* 64: 146–163.

Essock, Susan M., and Howard H. Goldman. 1995. "States' Embrace of Managed Mental Health Care."*Health Affairs* 14: 34–44.

Estroff, Sue E. 1981. *Making It Crazy: An Ethnography of Psychiatric Patients in an American Community.* Berkeley, CA: University of California Press.

Farber, Barry (ed.). 1983. *Stress and Burnout in Human Service Organizations.* New York: Pergamon Press.

Feldman, Sanford E., and Douglas W. Roblin. 1992. "Standards for Peer Evaluation: The Hospital Quality Assurance Committee." *American Journal of Public Health.* 82 (4): 525–527.

Fendell, Susan. 1998. "Privately Managed Mental Health: Shrinking Services." *International Journal of Mental Health* 27: 3–51.

Fennell, Mary L., and Jeffrey A. Alexander. 1993. "Perspectives on Organizational Change in The U.S. Medical Care Sector." *Annual Review of Sociology* 19: 89–112.

Filby, Mike P. 1992. "The Figures, the Personality and the Bums: Service Work and Sexuality." *Work, Employment and Society* 6: 23–42.

Finch, Ellen S., and Steven R. Krantz. 1991. "Low Burnout in a High Stress Setting: A Study of Staff Adaptation at Fountain House." *Psychosocial Rehabilitation Journal* 14: 15–26.

Findlay, William, Elizabeth Mutran, Rodney Zeitler, and Christina Randall. 1990. "Queues and Care: How Medical Residents Organize Their Work in a Busy Clinic." *Journal of Health and Social Behavior* 31: 292–305.

Fine, Gary A. 1984. "Negotiated Orders and Organizational Cultures." *Annual Review of Sociology* 19: 239–262.

———, and K. Sandstrom. 1993. "Ideology in Action: A Pragmatic Approach to a Contested Concept." *Sociological Theory* 11: 21–38.

Fineman, Stephen. 1993. *Emotions in Organizations.* London: Sage.

Fisher, William H., and Barbara Dickey. 1995. "Regional Variation in Service System Performance: Comparing the Perceptions of Key Stakeholders." *Journal of Mental Health Administration* 22: 68–76.

Fletcher, J. J. 1998. "Mental Health Nurses: Guardians of Ethics in Managed Care." *Journal of Psychosocial Nursing and Mental Health Services* 36: 34–37.

Flood, Ann Barry and Mary L. Fennell. 1995. "Through the Lens of Organizational Sociology: The Role of Organizational Theory and Research in Conceptualizing and Examining Our Health Care System." *Journal of Health and Social Behavior* (Special Issue): 154–169.

Flynn, Laurie. 1994. "Managed Care and Mental Illness." Pp. 203–210 in *Allies and Adversaries: The Impact of Managed Care in Mental Health Servivces,* edited by R. K. Schreter, S. S. Sharfstein, and C. A. Schreter. Washington, DC: American Psychological Association.

Foner, Nancy. 1995. *The Caregiving Dilemma: Work in an American Nursing Home.* Berkeley, CA: University of California Press.

Foucault, Michel. 1973. *The Birth of the Clinic: An Archaeology of Medical Perception.* New York: Vintage Books.

Frank, Richard G., Chris Koyanagi, and Thomas G. McGuire. 1997. "The Politics and Economics of Mental Health 'Parity' Laws." *Health Affairs* 16: 108–120.

Freidson, Eliot. 1984. "The Changing Nature of Professional Control." *Annual Review of Sociology* 10: 1–20.

———. 1986. *Professional Powers: A Study of the Institutionalization of Knowledge.* Chicago: University of Chicago Press.

———. 1989. *Medical Work in America: Essays in Health Care.* Chicago: University of Chicago Press.

Freund, Deborah A., and Robert E. Hurley. 1995. "Medicaid Managed Care: Contribution to Issues of Health Reform." *Annual Review of Public Health* 16: 473–495.

Furman, Rick. 2003. "Frameworks for Understanding Value Discrepancies and Ethical Dilemmas in Managed Mental Health for Social Work in the U.S." *International Social Work:* 46: 37–52.

Galambos, Colleen. 1999. "Resolving Ethical Conflicts in a Managed Health Care Environment." *Health and Social Work* 24: 191–198.

Galbraith, Jay. 1973. *Designing Complex Organizations.* Reading, MA: Addison Wesley.

Geertz, Clifford. 1983. *Local Knowledge: Further Essays in Intrepretative Anthropology.* New York: Basic Books.

Gervais, Karen G., Reinhard Priester, Dorthory E. Vawter, Kimberly K. Otte, and Mary M. Solberg. 1999. *Ethical Challenges in Managed Care: A Casebook.* Washington, DC: Georgetown University Press.

Glazer, Barney G., and Anselm L. Strauss. 1967. *The Discovery of Grounded Theory: Strategies for Qualitative Research.* Chicago: Aldine Publishing Co.

Glisson, C., and M. Durick. 1988. "Predictors of Job Satisfaction and Organizational Commitment in Human Service Organizations." *Administrative Science Quarterly* 33: 181.

Goffman, Irving. 1961. *Asylums.* New York: Anchor Books.

Goldman, Harold, J. P. Morrissey, and M. Susan Ridgely. 1994."Evaluating the Robert Wood Johnson Foundation Program on Chronic Mental Illness." *The Milibank Quarterly* 72: 37–48.

Golembiewski, Robert T., Richard Hilles, and Rick Daly. 1987. "Some Effects of Multiple OD Interventions on Burnout and Worksite Features." *Journal of Applied Behavioral Science* 23: 295–313.

———, Robert A. Boudreau, Robert F. Munzenrider, and Huaping Luo. 1996. *Global Burnout: A Worldwide Pandemic Explored by the Phase Model.* Greenwich, CT: JAI Press.

Goldin, Carol S. 1990. "Stigma, Biomedical Efficacy, and Institutional Control." *Social Science and Medicine* 30: 895–900.

Goll, Irene and Gerald Zeitz. 1991. "Conceptualizing and Measuring Corporate Ideology." *Organization Studies* 12: 191–207.

Gowdy, Elizabeth and Charles A. Rapp. 1989. "Managerial Behavior: The Common Denominators of Effective Community Based Programs." *Psychosocial Rehabilitation Journal* 13: 31–51.

Greenspan, S., and M. Cerreto. 1989. "Normalization, Deinstituitonalization, and the Limits of Research." *American Psychologist* 44: 448–449.

Gregory, Kathleen. 1983. "Native-view Paradigms: Multiple Cultures and Culture Conflicts in Organizations." *Administrative Science Quarterly* 28: 359–376.

Griffiths, Lesley and David Hughes. 1999. "Talking Contracts and Taking Care: Managers and Professionals in the British National Service Internal Market." *Social Science and Medicine:* 44: 1–13.

Grob, Gerald N. 1994. *The Mad Among Us: A History of Care of America's Mentally Ill.* New York: The Free Press.

Gudeman, Jon E. 1988. "The Evolution of a Public Psychiatric Hospital and Its System of Care." Pp. 25–32 in *Serving the Chronically Mentally Ill in an Urban Setting.* New Directions for Mental Health Services, No. 39, edited by M. F. Shore and J. E. Gudeman. San Francisco: Jossey-Bass.

Guy, Mary E. 1985. *Professionals in Organizations: Debunking a Myth.* New York: Praeger.

Hafferty, Frederic W., and Donald W. Light. 1995. "Professional Dynamics and the Changing Nature of Medical Work." *Journal of Health and Social Behavior* (Special Issue) 154–167.

———, and Frederic D. Wolinsky, 1991. "Conflicting Characterizations of Professional Dominance." *Current Research in Occupations and Professions* 6: 225–249.

Hall, Peter. 1986. *Dimensions of Work.* Beverly Hills, CA: Sage Publications.

Halpern, Sydney A. 1992. "Dynamics of Professional Control: Internal Coalitions and Crossprofessional Boundaries." *American Journal of Sociology* 97: 994–1021.

Handy, Jocelyn. 1988. "Theoretical and Methodological Problems within Occupational Stress and Burnout Research." *Human Relations* 41: 351–369.

Hannan, Michael T., and John Freeman. 1977. "The Population Ecology of Organizations." *American Journal of Sociology* 82: 929–964.

Hanson, K. W. and H. A. Huskamp. 2001. "State Health Care Reform: Behavioral Health Services Under Medicaid Managed Care." *Psychiatric Services* 52 (4): 447–450.

Harris, Maxine and Helen C. Bergman. 1987. "Case Management with the Chronically Mentally Ill: A Clinical Perspective." *American Journal of Orthopsychiatry* 57: 296–302.

Hasenfeld, Yeheskel (ed.). 1992. *Human Services as Complex Organizations.* Newbury Park, CA: Sage.

——— and Mark A. Chesler. 1989. "Client Empowerment and the Human Services: Personal and Professional Agendas." *Human Relations* 25: 499–521.

Hattersley, John. 1991. "The Future of Normalization." Pp. 1–11 in *Mental Handicap: Social Science Perspectives,* edited by S. Baldwin and J. Hattersley. New York: Routledge.

Haug, Marie R. 1994. "Elderly Patients, Caregivers and Physicians: Theory and Research in Health Care Triads." *Journal of Health and Social Behavior* 35: 1–12.

Hawthorne, William and Richard Hough. 1997. "Integrated Services for Long-term Care." Pp. 205–206 in *Managed Mental Health Care in the Public Sector,* edited by K. Minkoff and D. Pollack. Amsterdam, The Netherlands: Harwood Academic Publishers.

Heaney, C. A., and A. C. Burke. 1995. "Ideologies of Care in Community Residential Services: What Do Caregivers Believe?" *Community Mental Health Journal* 31: 449–462.

Heithoff, Kim A., and Kathleen N. Lohr (editors). 1990. *Effectiveness and Outcomes in Health Care.* Washington, DC: National Academy Press.

Hermann, Richard C., Stephen H. Left, Heather R. Palmer, Dawei Yang, Terri Teller, Scott Provost, Chet Jakubiak, and Jeff Chan. 2000. "Quality Measures for Mental Health Care: Results from a National Inventory." *Medical Care Research and Review* 57: 136–55.

Herron, William. 1997. "Restructuring Managed Mental Health Care." Pp. 217–231 in *The Impact of Managed Care on the Practice of Psychotherapy,* edited by R. M. Alperin and D. G. Phillips. New York: Brunner/Mazel Publishers.

Heydeband, Wolf. 1990. "The Technocratic Organization of Academic Work." Pp. 271–320 in *Structures of Power and Constraint,* edited by C. Calhoun, M. W. Meyer and W. R. Scott. Cambridge: Cambridge University Press.

Himmelweit, Susan. 1999. "Caring Labor." Pp. 27–38 in *Emotional Labor in the Service Economy: Special Issues of The Annals of the American Academy of Political and Social Science. Vol 56,* edited by Ronnie J. Steinberg and Deborah M. Figard. Thousands Oaks, CA: Sage.

Hochschild, Arlie Russell. 1983. *The Managed Heart: Commercialization of Human Feeling.* Berkeley: University of California Press.

———. 1989. "Reply to Cas Wouter's Essay on *The Managed Heart.*" *Theory, Culture and Society* 6: 439–445.

———. 1990. "Ideology and Emotion Management: A Perspective and Path for Future Research." Pp. 117–142 in *Research Agendas in the Sociology of Emotions*, edited by Theodore D. Kemper. Albany, NY: State University of New York Press.

Hoff, Timothy and David P. MCaffrey. 1996. "Adapting, Resisting, and Negotiating: How Physicians Cope with Organizational and Economic Change." *Work and Occupations:* 23: 165–189.

———, Winthrop F. Whitcomb, and John R. Nelson. 2002. "Thriving and Surviving in a New Medical Career: The Case of Hospital Practice." *Journal of Health and Social Behavior* 43: 15–42.

Hoge, M. A., L. Davidson, E. Griffith, W. H. Sledge, and R. A. Howenstine. 1994. "Defining Managed Care in Public-Sector Psychiatry." *Hospital and Community Psychiatry* 45: 1085–1089.

Holland, Thomas P., Andrew Konick, William Buffum, Milko Smith, and Marcia Petcher. 1981. "Institutional Structure and Patient Outcomes." *Journal of Health and Social Behavior* 22: 433–444.

Holstein, James A. 1992. "Producing People: Descriptive Practice in Social Work." *Current Research in Occupations and Professions* 7: 23–39.

Horwitz, Allan V. 1982. *The Social Control of Mental Illness.* New York: Academic Press.

———. 1987. "Help-Seeking Processes and Mental Health Services." *Improving Mental Health Services: What the Social Sciences Can Tell Us*, edited by D. Mechanic. San Francisco: Jossey-Bass.

———. 2002. *Creating Mental Illness.* Chicago: University of Chicago Press.

Hoyt, Michael F., and Carol S. Austad. 1992. "Psychotherapy in a Staff Model Health Maintenance Organization: Providing and Assuring Quality Care in the Future." *Psychotherapy* 29: 119–128.

Hurley, R. E. 1997. "Managed Care Research: Moving Beyond Incremental Thinking." *Health Services Research* 32: 679–691.

Igelhart, John K. 1996. "Managed Care and Mental Health." *The New England Journal of Medicine* 334: 131–135.

Ingleby, David. 1982. "The Social Construction of Mental Illness." Pp. 123–143 in *The Problem of Medical Knowledge: Examining the Social Construction of Medicine*, edited by Peter Wright and Andrew Treacher. Edinburgh, UK: Edinburgh University Press.

Institite of Medicine. 1997. *Managing Managed Care: Quality Improvement in Behavioral Health.* Washington, DC: National Academy Press.

Jackson, Susan E., Richard A. Schwab, and Randall S. Schuler. 1986. "Toward an Understanding of the Burnout Phenomenon." *Journal of Applied Psychology* 71: 630–640.

Jacobson, Nora and Dianne Greenley. 2001. "What Is Recovery? A Conceptual Model and Explication." *Psychiatric Services* 52 (4): 482–485.

James, Nicky. 1989. "Emotional Labour: Skill and Work in the Regulation of Feelings. *Sociological Review* 37: 15–42.

Jayaratne, Scinika and Wayne A. Chess. 1983. "Job Satisfaction and Burnout in Social Work. Pp. 129–141 in *Stress and Burnout in Human Service Organizations*, edited by B. Farber. New York: Pergamon Press.

Jensen, Gail A., Michael A. Morrisey, Shannon Gaffney, and Derek K. Liston. 1997. "The New Dominance of Managed Care: Insurance Trends in the 1990s." *Health Affairs* 16: 125–135.

———, Kathryn Roos, Russell P. D. Burten, and Maria Bulycheva. 1998. "Mental

Health Insurance in the 1990s: Are Employers Offering Less for More?" *Health Affairs* 17: 201–208.

Jerrell, Jeanette M., and Judith K. Larson. 1984. "Policy Shifts and Organizational Adaptation: A Review of Current Developments." *Community Mental Health Journal* 20: 282–293.

————, and William A. Hargreaves. 1989. Community Program Philosophy Scale (CPPS): Preliminary Report. Institute for Mental Health. Services Research, Berkeley, California.

Kahn, William. 1993. "Caring for the Caregivers: Patterns of Organizational Caregiving." *Administrative Science Quarterly* 38: 539–563.

Karasek, Robert and Tores Theorell. 1990. *Health Work: Stress, Productivity, and the Reconstruction of Working Life.* New York: Basic Books.

Kessler, Ronald C., and Shanyang Zhao. 1999. "The Prevalence of Mental Illness." Pp. 58–78 in *A Handbook for the Study of Mental Health,* edited by A. V. Horwitz and T. L. Scheid. Cambridge: Cambridge University Press.

Kesey, Ken. 1962. *One Flew Over the Cuckoo's Nest.* New York: Penguin.

Keyes, Corey L. M. 2002. "The Mental Health Continuum: From Languishing to Flourishing in Life." *Journal of Health and Social Behavior* 43: 207–22.

Kihlstrom, Lucy C. 1997. "Characteristics and Growth of Managed Behavioral Health Care Firms." *Health Affairs* 16: 127–130.

Kirk, Stuart A. and Herb Kutchins. 1992. *The Selling of the DSM: The Rhetoric of Science in Psychiatry,* Hawthorne, NY: Aldine de Gruyter.

Kirk, Stuart A., Gary F. Loeske, and Randi Koeske. 1993. "Changes in Health and Job Attitudes of Case Managers Providing Intensive Services." *Hospital and Community Psychiatry* 44: 168–173.

Kirschner, Suzane R., and William S. Lachiotte. 2001. "Managing Managed Care: Habitus, Hysteresis and the End(s) of Psychotherapy." *Culture and Medicine in Psychiatry* 25: 441–456.

Kleinman, Arthur. 1988. *The Illness Narratives.* New York: Basic Books.

Koeske, Gary F., and Stuart A. Kirk. 1995. "The Effect of Characteristics of Human Service Workers on Subsequent Moral and Turnover." *Administration in Social Work* 19: 15–31.

Lake, Eileen T. 1998. "Advances in Understanding and Predicting Nurse Turnover." *Research in the Sociology of Health Care* 15: 147–171.

Lamb, Richard H. 1982. *Treating the Long Term Mentally Ill.* San Francisco: Jossey-Bass.

Lang, Claire L. 1981. "Good Cases-Bad Cases: Client Selection and Professional Prerogative in a Community Mental Health Center." *Urban Life* 10: 289–309.

Langton, Patricia A. 1991. "Competing Occupational Ideologies, Identities, and the Practice of Nurse-Midwifery." *Current Perspectives in Occupations and Professions* 6: 149–177.

LaRoche, Martin J., and Castellano Turner. 2002. "At the Crossroads: Managed Mental Health Care, the Ethics Code, and Ethnic Minorities." *Cultural Diversity and Ethnic Minority Psychology.* 2002: 187–198.

Larson, Magali Sarfatti. 1977. *The Rise of Professionalism.* Berkeley, CA: University of California Press.

Latack, Janina C. 1986. "Coping With Job Stress: Measures and Future Directions in Scale Development." *Journal of Applied Psychology* 71: 377–385.

Lazarus, Jeremy and David Pollack. 1997. "Ethical Aspects of Public Sector Managed Care." Pp. 25–36 in *Managed Mental Health in the Public Sector,* edited by K. Minkoff and D. Pollack. Amsterdam, The Netherlands: Harwood Academic Publishers.

Lefley, Harriet P. 1984. "Delivering Mental Health Services Across Cultures." Pp. 135–171 in *Mental Health Services: The Cross Cultural Context,* edited by Pederson, P., Satorius, N., Marsella, A. J. Beverly Hills: Sage.

Lehman, Anthony. 1999. "Quality of Care in Mental Health: The Case of Schizophrenia." *Health Affairs* 18: 22–36.

Leidner, Robin. 1993. *Fast Food, Fast Talk: Service Work and the Routinization of Everyday Life.* Berkeley, CA: University of California Press.

Leiter, Michael P. 1988. "Burnout as a Function of Communication Patterns: A Study of a Multidisciplinary Treatment Team." *Group and Organization Studies* 13: 111–128.

Leiter, Michael P. 1990. "The Impact of Family Resources, Control, Coping, and Skill Utilization on the Development of Burnout: A Longitudinal Study." *Human Relations* 43: 1067- 1083.

Leiter, Michael P. 1991. "Coping Patterns in Predictors of Burnout: The Function of Control and Escapist Coping Patterns." *Journal of Organizational Behavior* 12: 123–144.

Levitt, Brian and James G. March. 1998. "Organizational Learning" *Annual Review of Sociology* 14: 319–340.

Light, Donald W. 1997. "The Rhetorics and Realities of Community Health Care: The Limits of Countervailing Powers to Meet the Health Care Needs of the Twenty-first Century." *Journal of Health Politics, Policy and Law* 22: 106–145.

Light, Donald W. 2001. "Cost Containment and the Backdraft of Competition Policies." *International Journal of Health Services* 31: 681–708.

Light, Donald, Mary L. Fennell and Kristine M. Witkowski. 1995. "The Effects of Hospital Characteristics and Radical Organizational Change in the Relative Standing of Health Care Professions." *Journal of Health and Social Behavior* 36: 151–167.

Light, Donald. 1991. "Social Control and the American Health Care System." Pp. 456–472 in *Handbook of Medical Sociology,* 4e, edited by H. E. Freeman and S. Levine. Englewood Cliffs, NJ: Prentice-Hall.

Link, Bruce G. 1987. "Understanding Labeling Effects in the Area of Mental Disorder." *American Sociological Review* 47: 202–15.

Link, Bruce G., and Jo Phelan. 1995. "Social Conditions as Fundamental Causes of Disease." *Journal of Health and Social Behavior* (Special Issue): 80–94.

Lively, Kathryn. 2002. "Client Contact and Emotional Labor: Upsetting the Balance and Evening the Field." *Work and Occupations,* 29: 198–225.

Locke, Karen. 1996. "A Funny Thing Happened! The Management of Consumer Emotions in Service Encounters." *Organization Science* 7: 40–59.

Ludwig, Karen Joan and David A. Molz. 1997. "Time-Sensitive Treatment in Community Mental Health Settings." Pp. 257–269 in *Managed Mental Health Care in the Public Sector,* edited by K. Minkoff and D. Pollack. Amsterdam, The Netherlands: Harwood Academic Publishers.

Luhrmann, T. M. 2000. *Of Two Minds: The Growing Disorder in American Psychiatry.* New York: Alfred Knopf.

Lupton, Deborah. 1997. "Doctors and the Medical Profession." *Sociology of Health and Illness* 19: 480–497.

Lurie, N. 1997. "Studying Access to Care in Managed Care Environments." *Health Services Research* 32: 691–701.

MacDonald, Don. 1991. "Philosophies That Underlie Models of Mental Health Counseling: More Than Meets the Eye." *Journal of Mental Health Counseling* 13: 379–392.

Mackey, Richard A., Mitchell Burek, and Susan Charkoudian. 1987. "The Relationship of Theory to Clinical Practice." *Clinical Social Work Journal* 15: 368–383.

Magaro, Peter A., Robert Gripp, and David J. McDowell. 1978. *The Mental Health Industry: A Cultural Phenomenon.* New York: John Wiley and Sons.

Manderscheid, Ronald W., Marilyn J. Henderson, Michael J. Witkin, and Joanne E. Atay. 1999. "Contemporary Mental Health Systems and Managed Care." Pp. 412–426 in *A Handbook for the Study of Mental Health,* edited by A. V. Horwitz and T. L. Scheid. Cambridge: Cambridge University Press.

———. 2000. "The U. S. Mental Health System of the 1990s: The Challenges of Managed Care." *International Journal of Law and Psychiatry.* 23: 245–59.

Mannhein, Karl. 1936. *Ideology and Utopia: An Introduction to the Sociology of Knowledge.* New York: Harcourt Brace Publishers.

Markowitz, Fred E. 2001. "Modeling Processes in Recovering from Mental Illness: Relationships Between Symptoms, Life Satisfaction, and Self Concept." *Journal of Health and Social Behavior* 42: 64–79.

Martin, Joanne. 1992. *Cultures in Organizations: Three Perspectives.* New York: Oxford.

Martin, Lawrence and Peter M. Kettner. 1997. "Performance Measurement: The New Accountability." *Administration in Social Work* 21: 17–29.

Maslach, Christina. 1982. *Burnout: The Cost of Caring.* Englewood Cliffs, NJ: Prentice-Hall.

———, and S. E. Jackson. 1981. "The Measurement of Experienced Burnout." *Journal of Occupational Behavior* 2: 99–113.

McFarland, Benson. 2001. "Assessments, Interventions, and Outcomes: Who Cares?" *Community Mental Health Journal* 37: 93–5.

McLean, Athena Helen. 2000. "From Ex-Patient Alternatives to Consumer Options: Consequences of Consumerism For Psychiatric Consumers and the Ex-Patient Movement." *Sociology of Health and Illness* 30: 821–847.

McNeely, Robert L. 1983. "Organizational Patterns and Work Satisfaction in a Comprehensive Human Service Agency: An Empirical Test." *Human Relations* 36: 957–972.

———. 1992. "Job Satisfaction in the Public Social Services: Perspectives on Structure, Situation Factors, Gender, and Ethnicity." Pp. 224–255 in *Human Services as Complex Organizations,* edited by Y. Hasenfeld. Newbury Park: Sage.

Mechanic, David. 1976. *The Growth of Bureaucratic Medicine.* New York: John Wiley.

———. 1986. "The Challenge of Chronic Mental Illness: A Retrospective and Prospective View." *Hospital and Community Psychiatry* 37: 891–896.

———. 1989. "Medical Sociology: Some Tension Among Theory, Method and Substance." *Journal of Health and Social Behavior* 30: 147–160.

———. 1994. "Establishing Mental Health Priorities." *The Milibank Quarterly* 72: 501–514.

———. 1999. *Mental Health and Social Policy: The Emergence of Managed Care.* Boston: Allyn and Bacon.

———— and David Rochefort. 1990. "Deinstitutionalization: An Appraisal of Reform." *Annual Review of Sociology* 16: 301–327.

———— and Mark Schlesinger. 1993. "Challenges for Managed Competition From Chronic Illness." *Health Affairs* (Supplement) 12: 123–137.

————. 1996. "The Impact of Managed Care on Patients' Trust in Medical Care and Their Physicians." *JAMA* 275 (21): 1693–1697.

————, and Donna McAlpine. 1995. "Management of Mental Health and Substance Abuse Services: State of the Art and Early Results." *The Milibank Quarterly* 73: 19–55.

Mechanic, David and Donna McAlpine. 1999. "Mission Unfulfilled: Potholes on the Road to Mental Health Parity." *Health Affairs* 18: 7–21.

Meyer, Marshall W. 1990. "The Weberian Tradition in Organizational Research." Pp. 191–215 in *Structures of Power and Constraint*, edited by C. Calhoun, M. W. Meyer, and W. R. Scott. Cambridge: Cambridge University Press.

Meyer, John W. and Brian Rowan. 1983. "The Structure of Educational Organizations." Pp. 71–97. *Organizational Environments: Ritual and Rationality*. Beverly Hills: Sage.

————, and W. Richard Scott. 1983. *Organizational Environments: Ritual and Rationality.* Beverly Hills: Sage.

Meyerson, Debra E. 1991. "Normal Ambiguity: A Glimpse of an Occupational Culture." Pp. 131–156 in *Reframing Organizational Culture*, edited by P. J. Frost, L. F. Moore, M. R. Louis, C. Lundenberg, and J. Martin. Newbury Park, CA: Sage.

————. 1994. "Interpretations of Stress in Institutions: The Cultural Production of Ambiguity and Burnout." *Administrative Science Quarterly* 39: 628–653.

Michels, Robert and Peter M. Marzuk. 1993. "Progress in Psychiatry." *The New England Journal of Medicine* 329: 552–560.

Miller, Robert H., and Harold S. Luft. 1997. "Does Managed Care Lead to Better or Worse Quality of Care?" *Health Affairs* 16: 7–25.

Millman, Marcia. 1977. *The Unkindest Cut: Life in the Backrooms of Medicine.* New York: Morrow Quill Paperbacks.

Minkoff, Debra C. 1993. "The Organization of Survival: Women's and Racial-Ethnic Voluntarist and Activist Organizations, 1955–1985." *Social Forces* 71: 887–908.

Minkoff, Kenneth. 1997. "Public Sector Managed Care and Community Mental Health Ideology." Pp. 13–22 in *Managed Mental Health in the Public Sector*, edited by K. Minkoff and D. Pollack. Amsterdam, The Netherlands: Harwood Academic Publishers.

———— and David Pollack (eds.). 1997. *Managed Mental Health in the Public Sector.* Amsterdam, The Netherlands: Harwood Academic Publishers.

Mirowsky, John and Catherine E. Ross. 1989. "Psychiatric Diagnosis as Reified Measurement." *Journal of Health and Social Behavior* 30: 11–25.

————. 2002. "Measurement in Human Science." *Journal of Health and Social Behavior* 43: 152–170.

Mishler, Elliot G. 1989. "Critical Perspectives on the Biomedical Model." Pp. 153–166 in *Perspectives in Medical Sociology*, edited by Phil Brown. Belmont, CA: Wadsworth Publishing.

Mizrahi, Terry. 1986. *Getting Rid of Patients: Contradictions in the Socialization of Physicians.* New Brunswick, NJ: Rutgers University Press.

Moffic, H. Steven. 1997. *The Ethical Way: Challenges and Solutions for Managed Behavioral Healthcare.* San Francisco: Jossey-Bass Publications.

Moore, Wilbert E. 1970. *The Professions: Roles and Rules.* New York: Russell Sage Foundation.

Moos, Rudolf H. 1974. *Evaluating Treatment Environments: A Social Ecological Approach.* New York: John Wiley and Sons.

Morgan, Gareth. 1986. *Images of Organizations.* Beverly Hills, CA: Sage.

Morris, J. Andrew and Daniel C. Feldman. 1996. "The Dimensions, Antecedents, and Consequences of Emotional Labor." *Academy of Management Review* 21: 986–1010.

Morrissey, Joseph P. 1999. "Integrating Service Delivery Systems for Persons with Severe Mental Illness." Pp. 449–466 in *A Handbook for the Study of Mental Health,* edited by A. V. Horwitz and T. L. Scheid. Cambridge: Cambridge University Press.

———, and Michael C. Calloway. 1994. "Local Mental Health Authorities and Service System Change: Evidence From the Robert Wood Johnson Foundation Program on Chronic Mental Illness." *The Milibank Quarterly* 72: 49–80.

———, Howard H. Goldman, and Lorraine V. Klerman. 1980. *The Enduring Asylum.* New York: Grune and Stratton.

———, Mark Tausig, and Michael L. Linsday. 1984. "Interorganizational Networks in Mental Health Services. Assessing Community Programs for the Chronically Mentally Ill." Presented at the Workshop for Organizations and Mental Health, National Institute of Mental Health. September 17–18.

Motowidlo, Stephen J., John S. Packard, and Michael Manning. 1986. "Occupational Stress: Its Causes and Consequences for Job Performance." *Journal of Applied Psychology* 71: 618–629.

Mumby, Dennis K. 1988. *Communication and Power in Organizations: Discourse, Ideology, and Domination.* Norwood, NJ: Ablex Publishing Corp.

National Alliance for the Mentally Ill. 1997. "Stand and Deliver: Action Call to a Failing Industry." See http://www.nami.org.

———. 2003. "National Managed Care Patient Bill of Rights." See http://www.nami.org.

National Center for Health Statistics. 1992. Advance Data No. 218, September 16.

National Council on Disability. 2002. "The Well-Being of Our Nation: An Intergenerational Vision of Effective Mental Health Services and Supports." Washington, DC. See http://www.ncd.org.

Neugeboren, Jay. 1997. *Imaging Robert: My Brother, Madness and Survival.* New York: Henry Holt and Company.

———. 1999. *Transforming Madness: New Lives for People Living with Mental Illness.* Berkeley, CA: University of California Press.

Nijsmans, Mia. 1991. "Professional Cultures and Organizational Morality: An Ethnographic Account of a Therapeutic Organization." *British Journal of Sociology* 42: 1–19.

Oberlander, Lois B. 1990. "Work Satisfaction Among Community-Based Mental Health Service Providers: The Association Between Work Environment and Work Satisfaction." *Community Mental Health Journal* 26: 517–532.

O'Brien, R. M. 1991. "Correcting Measures of Relationship Between Aggregate Level Variables." Pp. 125–165 in *Sociological Methodology,* edited by P. V. Marsden. Oxford: Basil Blackwell.

182   References

O'Brien, Martin. 1994. "The Managed Heart Revisited: Health and Social Control." *Sociological Review* 42: 393–413.

O'Driscoll, Michael P. and Rosalind Evans. 1988. "Organizational Factors and Perceptions of Climate in Three Psychiatric Units." *Human Relations* 41: 371–388.

Ogles, Benjamin M., Steven C. Trout, D. Kevin Gillespie, and Kathleen S. Penkert. 1998. "Managed Care as a Platform for Cross-System Integration." *The Journal of Behavioral Health Services & Research* 25: 252–268.

Paine, Whiton Stewart. 1982. *Job Stress and Burnout: Research, Theory and Intervention Perspectives.* Beverly Hills, CA: Sage Publications.

Paulin, J. E. 1994. "Job Task and Organizational Predictors of Social worker Job Satisfaction Change: A Panel Study." *Administration in Social Work* 18: 21–38.

Paulson, R. 1992. "Advocacy and Empowerment: Mental Health Care in the Community." *Community Mental Health Journal* 28: 70–1.

Perrow, Charles. 1965. "Hospitals, Technology, Structure, and Goals." In *Handbook of Organizations,* edited by J. March. Chicago: Rand McNally.

Perruci, Robert. 1974. *Circles of Madness: On Being Insane and Institutionalized in America.* Englewood Cliffs, NJ: Prentice Hall.

Peterson, Christopher. 1999. "Psychological Approaches to Mental Illness." Pp. 104–120 in *A Handbook for the Study of Mental Health,* edited by A. V. Horwitz and T. L. Scheid. Cambridge: Cambridge University Press.

Peyrot, Mark. 1991. "Institutional and Organizational Dynamics in Community Based Drug Abuse Treatment." *Social Problems* 38: 20–33.

Pfohl, Stephan. J. 1978. *Predicting Dangerousness: The Social Construction of Psychiatric Reality.* Lexington, MA: Lexington Books.

Phillips, David G. 1997. "Legal and Ethical Issues in the Era of Managed Care." Pp. 171–184 in *The Impact of Managed Care on the Practice of Psychothrapy,* edited by R. M. Alperin and D. G. Phillips. New York: Brunner/Mazel Publishers.

Pines, Ayal and Maslach, Christina. 1978. "Characteristics of Staff Burnout in Mental Health Settings." *Hospital and Community Psychiatry* 29: 233–237.

Pittman, Deanna C. 1989. "Nursing Case Management: Holistic Care for the Deinstitutionalized Chronically Mentally Ill." *Journal of Psychosocial Nursing* 27: 23–27.

Pogrebin, Mark R., and Eric D. Poole. 1995. "Emotion Management: A Study of Police Response to Tragic Events." *Social Perspectives on Emotion* 3: 149–168.

Pollack, D., B. H. McFarland, R. A. George and R. H. Angell. 1994. "Prioritization of Mental Health Services in Oregon." *The Milibank Quarterly* 72: 515–550.

Powell, Walter W. 1991. "Expanding the Scope of Institutional Analysis." Pp. 183–203 in *The New Institutionalism in Organizational Analysis,* edited by W. W. Powell and P. J. DiMaggio. Chicago: University of Chicago Press.

———, and Paul J. DiMaggio (eds.). 1991. *The New Institutionalism in Organizational Analysis.* Chicago: University of Chicago Press.

Prager, Edward. 1986. "Bureaucracy's Impact on Decison Making in Long Term Care." *Health and Social Work* 11: 275–285.

Price, James L. 1989. "The Impact of Turnover on the Organization." *Work and Occupations* 6: 461–473.

Provan, Keith and H. Brinton Milward. 1995. "A Preliminary Theory of Interorganizational Network Effectiveness: A Comparative Study of Four Community Mental Health Systems." *Administrative Science Quarterly* 40: 1–33.

Pugliesi, Karen. 1999. "The Consequences of Emotional Labor: Effects on Work Stress, Job Satisfaction and Well Being." *Motivation and Emotion* 23: 125–154.

Rafaeli, Anat and Sutton, Robert. 1989. "The Expression of Emotion in Organizational Life." In *Research in Organizational Behavior*, edited by L. L Cummings and B. M. Staw, Vol 11: 1–42. Greenwich, CT: JAI Press.

Ragin, Charles C. 1999. "The Distinctiveness of Case-Oriented Research." *Health Services Research*. 34: 1137–51.

Reid, Y. S. Younson, N. Morant, E. Kulpers, G. Szmukler, G. Thornicroft, P. Bebbington, D. Prossier. 1999. "Explanations for Stress and Satisfaction in Mental Health Professionals: A Qualitative Study." *Social Psychiatry and Social Epidemiology*. 34: 301–308.

Rochefort, David. 1989. *Handbook on Mental Health Policy in the US*. New York: Greenwood Press.

Rodwin, Marc A. 1993. *Medicine, Money and Morals: Physicians' Conflicts of Interest*. New York: Oxford University Press.

Rose, Stephen P., and Bruce L. Black. 1985. *Advocacy and Empowerment: Mental Health Care in the Community*. Boston: Routledge and Kegan Paul.

Rosenberg, Morris. 1992. *The Unread Mind: Unraveling the Mystery of Madness*. New York: Lexington Books.

Rosenfield, Sarah. 1989. "Psychiatric Epidemiology: An Overview of Methods and Research Findings." Pp. 45–65 in *Handbook on Mental Health Policy in the U. S.*, edited by D. Rochefort. New York: Greenwood Press.

———. 1997. "Labeling Mental Illness: The Effects of Received Services and Perceived Stigma on Life Satisfaction." *American Sociological Review* 62: 660–672.

Rubin, Allen and Peter J. Johnson. 1984. "Direct Practice Interests of Entering MSW Students." *Journal of Education for Social Work* 20: 5–16.

Ryff, Carol D. 1989. "Happiness Is Everything, or Is It? Explorations on the Meaning of Psychological Well-Being." *Journal of Personality and Social Psychology* 57: 1069–1081.

Sabin, James E., and Norman Daniels. 2001. "Strengthening the Consumer in Managed Care: Part I. Can the Private Sector Meet the Public Sector Standard?" *Psychiatric Services* 52 (4): 461–465.

Salaman, Graeme. 1980. "Organizations as Constructors of Social Reality." Pp. 237–256 in G. Salaman and K. Thompson (eds.). *Control and Ideology in Organizations*. Cambridge, MA: MIT Press.

Salzer, Mark. 1999. "The Outcomes Measurement Movement and Mental Health Services Research." *Mental Health Services Research* 1 (1): 59–63.

Saylers, Michelle P., and Gary R. Bond. 2001. "An Exploratory Analysis of Racial Factors In Staff Burnout Among Assertive Community Treatment Workers." *Community Mental Health Journal*. 37: 393–404.

Saxton, Mary Jane, James S. Phillips, and Roger N. Blakeney. 1991. "Antecedents and Consequences of Emotional Exhaustion in the Airline Reservations Service Sector." *Human Relations* 44: 583–595.

Scanlon, Dennis P., Elizabeth Rolph, Charles Darby and Hilary Doty. 2000. "Are Managed Care Plans Organizing for Quality?" *Medical Care Research and Review* 57: 9–33.

Schatzman, Leonard and Anselm Strauss. 1973. *Field Research: Strategies for a Natural Sociology*. Englewood Cliffs, NJ: Prentice-Hall.

Schaubroeck, John and Deryl E. Merritt. 1997. "Divergent Effects of Job Control on Coping with Work Stressors: The Key Role of Self Efficacy." *Academy of Management Journal* 40: 738–754.

Scheff, Thomas J. 1984. *Being Mentally Ill: A Sociological Theory.* New York: Aldine Publishing Co.

Scheid, Teresa. 1993. "Controller and Controlled: An Analysis of Participant Constructions of Outpatient Commitment." *Sociology of Health and Illness.* 15: 179–193.

———. 1994. "An Explication of Treatment Ideology Among Mental Health Care Providers." *Sociology of Health and Illness* 16: 668–693.

———, and Anne Mayer. 1995. "Holding on to Success: A Case Study in Mental Health Care Reform." *The Journal of Mental Health Administration* 22: 29–37.

———. 1999a. "Emotional Labor and Burnout Among Mental Health Professionals." *Perspectives on Social Problems* 11: 169–193.

———. 1999b. "Mental Health Systems and Policy." Pp. 377–391 in *A Handbook for the Study of Mental Health,* edited by A. V. Horwitz and T. L. Scheid. Cambridge: Cambridge University Press.

———. 2002. "Managed Care, Managed Dollars, Managed Providers: Ethical Dilemmas in Mental Health Care." *Healthcare Ethics Forum* 14:99–118.

———, and James R. Greenley. 1997. "Evaluations of Organizational Effectiveness in Mental Health Care Programs." *Journal of Health and Social Behavior* 38: 403–26.

———, Elizabeth Fayram, and Vivian Littlefield. 1998. "Work Experiences of Mental Health Care Providers: Professional and Organizational Determinants of Burnout and Satisfaction." *Research in the Sociology of Health Care* 15: 51–76.

Scheid-Cook, Teresa L. 1988. "Mitigating Organizational Contradictions: The Role of Mediatory Myths." *The Journal of Applied Behavioral Science* 24: 161–171.

———. 1990. "Ritual Conformity and Organizational Control: Loose-coupling or Professionalization?" *The Journal of Applied Behavioral Science* 26: 183–199.

———. 1991. "Outpatient Commitment as Both Social Control and Least Restrictive Alternative." *Sociological Quarterly* 32: 433–460.

———. 1992. "Organizational Enactments and Conformity to Environmental Prescriptions." *Human Relations* 45: 537–554.

Schinnar, A. P., E. Kamis-Gould, N. Dulucia, and A. B. Rothbard 1990. "Organizational Determinants of Efficiency and Effectiveness in Mental Health Partial Care Programs." *Health Services Research* 25: 387–420.

Schlesinger, Mark J. 1995. "Ethical Issues in Policy Advocacy." *Health Affairs* 14: 23–29.

——— and Bradford H. Gray. 1999. "Institutional Change and Its Consequences for the Delivery of Mental Health Services." Pp. 427–448 in *A Handbook for the Study of Mental Health,* edited by A. V. Horwitz and T. L. Scheid. Cambridge: Cambridge University Press.

———, Bradford H. Gray, and Krista M. Perreira. 1997. "Medical Professionalism Under Managed Care: The Pros and Cons of Utilization Review." *Health Affairs* 16 (1): 106–124.

Schreter, Robert, Steven S. Sharfstein, and Carol A. Schreter. 1994. *Allies and Adversaries: The Impact of Managed Care on Mental Health Services.* Washington, DC: American Psychiatric Press.

Schulz, Rockwell, and James R. Greenley. 1995. *Innovating in Community Mental Health*. Westport, CT: Praeger.

———, James R. Greenley, and Roger Brown. 1995. "Organization, Management, and Client Effects on Staff Burnout in Care for Persons with Severe Mental Illness." *Journal of Health and Social Behavior* 36: 333–345.

Schwalbe, Michael L. 1986. *The Psychosocial Consequences of Natural and Alienated Labor*. Albany, NY: State University of New York Press.

Scott, R. A., L. A. Aiken, D. Mechanic, and J. Moravcsik. 1995. "Organizational Aspects of Caring." *The Milibank Quarterly* 73: 77–93.

Scott, W. Richard. 1983. "Health Care Organizations in the 1980's: The Convergence of Public and Professional Control Systems." Pp. 99–114 in *Organizational Environments*, edited by J. W. Meyer and W. R. Scott. Beverly Hills, CA: Sage.

———. 1985. "Conflicting Levels of Rationality: Regulators, Managers, and Professionals in the Medical Care Sector." *The Journal of Health Administration Education* 3: 113–131.

———. 1992. *Organizations: Rational, Natural, and Open Systems*, 3rd ed. Englewood Cliffs, NJ: Prentice-Hall.

———. 1993. "The Organization of Medical Care Services: Toward an Integrated Theoretical Model." *Medical Care Review* 50: 271–303.

———. 1995. *Institutions and Organizations*. Thousand Oaks, CA: Sage Publications.

——— and J. C. Lammers. 1985. "Trends in Occupations in the Medical Care and Mental Health Sectors." *Medical Care Review* 42: 37–76.

——— and J. W. Meyer. 1991. "The Organization of Societal Sectors: Propositions and Early Evidence." Pp. 108–140 in *The New Institutionalism in Organizational Analysis*, edited by W. W. Powell and P. J. DiMaggio. Chicago: University of Chicago Press.

———, Martin Ruef, Peter Mendel, and Carol A. Caroneer. 2000. *Institutional Change and Organizational Transformation of the Healthcare Field*. Chicago: University of Chicago Press.

Scull, Andrew. 1977. *Decarceration: Community Treatment and the Deviant*. Englewood Cliffs, NJ: Prentice-Hall.

Shadish, William R., Arthur J. Lurigio, and Don A. Lewis. 1989. "After Deinstitutionalism: The Present and Future of Mental Health Long-term Policy." *Journal of Social Issues* 45: 1–15.

Shore, Miles F., and Allan Biegel. 1996. "The Challenges Posed by Managed Behavioral Health Care." *The Milibank Quarterly* 73: 77–93.

Shortell, S. M. 1997. "Managed Care: Achieving the Benefits, Negating the Harm." *Health Services Research* 32: 557–560.

Siegler, Mirian and Humphry Osmond. 1974. *Models of Madness, Models of Medicine*. New York: Macmillan.

Smith, Pam. 1999. "Emotional Labor." *Soundings* 11: 14–19.

———. 1992. *The Emotional Labor of Nursing: How Nurses Care*. Basingstoke: Macmillan.

Soderfeldt, B. and M. Soderfeldt, C. Muntaner, P. O'campo, L. Warj, and C. Ohlsom. 1996. "Psychosocial Work Environment in Human Service Organizations: A Conceptual Analysis and Development of the Demand-Control Model." *Social Science and Medicine* 42: 1217–1226.

Spector, Paul E. 1983. "Measurement of Human Staff Satisfaction." *American Journal of Community Psychology* 13: 693–704.

Stamps, P. L., E. B. Piedmont, D. B. Slavitt, and A. M. Haase. 1978. "Measurement of Work Satisfaction among Health Professionals." *Medical Care* 16: 337–352.

Starr, Paul. 1982. *The Social Transformation of American Medicine*. New York: Basic Books.

Starrin, Bengt, Gerry Larsson, and Sven Styrborn. 1991. "A Review and Critique of Psychological Approaches to the Burn-out Phenomenon." *Scandinavian Journal of Caring Sciences* 4: 83–91.

Steinberg, Ronnie J., and Deborah M. Figard (eds.). 1999. "Introduction." *Emotional Labor in the Service Economy: Special Issue of The Annals of the American Academy of Political and Social Science*. Vol 561. Thousand Oaks, CA: Sage.

Stenross, Barbara and Sheryl Kleinman. 1989. "The Highs and Lows of Emotional Labor: Detectives' Encounters with Criminals and Victims." *Journal of Contemporary Ethnography* 17: 435–452.

Stern, Robert and Kenneth Minkoff. 1979. "Paradoxes in Programming for Chronic Patients in a Community Clinic." *Hospital and Community Psychiatry* 30: 613–617.

Strauss, Anselm L. 1987. *Qualitative Analysis for Social Scientists*. Cambridge: Cambridge University Press.

———, and Juliet Corbin. 1990. *Basics of Qualitative Research: Grounded Theory Procedures and Techniques*. Newbury Park, CA: Sage.

Strauss, Anselm, Leonard Schatzman, Rue Burcher, Danuta Ehrlich and Melvin Sabshin. 1964. *Psychiatric Ideologies and Institutions*. London: The Free Press.

———, Shizuko Fagerhaugh, Barbara Suczek, and Carolyn Wiener. 1985. *Social Organization of Medical Work*. Chicago: University of Chicago Press.

Stroup, T. Scott and Robert A. Dorwart. 1997. "Overview of Public Sector Managed Mental Health Care." Pp. 1–12 in *Managed Mental Health Care in the Public Sector*, edited by K. Minkoff and D. Pollack. The Netherlands: Harwood Academic Publishers.

Strout, Margaret. 1998. "Impact of Medicaid Managed Mental Health Care on the Delivery of Services in a Rural State: A NAMI Perspective." *Psychiatric Services* 49 (7): 961–963.

Susman, Joan. 1994. "Disability, Stigma and Deviance." *Social Science and Medicine* 38: 15–22.

Sutton, Robert L. 1991. "Maintaining Norms about Expressed Emotions: The Case of Bill Collectors." *Administrative Science Quarterly* 36: 245–268.

Szasz, Thomas S. 1963. *Law, Liberty and Psychiatry: An Inquirty into the Social Uses of Mental Health Practices*. New York: Macmillan.

———. 1984. *The Therapeutic State: Psychiatry in the Mirror of Current Events*. Buffalo, NY: Prometheus.

Szivos, S. E., and E. Travers. 1988. "Consciousness Raising Among Mentally Handicapped People: A Critique of the Implications of Normalization." *Human Relations* 41: 641–653.

Teisberg, Elizabeth Olmsted, Michael E. Porter, and Gregory B. Brown. 1994. "Making Competition in Health Care Work." *Harvard Business Review* 72: 131–141.

Teram, Eli. 1991. "Interdisciplinary Teams and the Control of Clients: A Socio-Technical Perspective." *Human Relations* 44: 343–356.

Tessler, Ronald and Howard Goldman. 1982. *The Chronically Mentally Ill: Assessing Community Suport Programs*. Cambridge, MA: Ballinger.

Thoits, Peggy A. 1990. "Emotional Deviance: Research Agendas." Pp. 180–203 in *Research Agendas in the Sociology of Emotions*, edited by Theodore D. Kemper. Albany, NY: State University of New York Press.

————. 1991. "On Merging Identity Theory and Stress Research." *Social Psychology Quarterly* 54: 101–112.

Thornquist, Eline. 1994. "Profession and Lifeworld: Separate Worlds." *Social Science and Medicine* 39: 701–713.

Thompson, Kenneth. 1980. "Organizations as Constructors of Social Reality." Pp. 216–236 in *Control and Ideology in Organizations*, edited by G. Salamon and K. Thompson. Cambridge, MA: MIT Press.

Thorton, Patricia I. 1992. "The Relation of Coping, Appraisal, and Burnout in Mental Health Workers." *The Journal of Psychology* 126: 261–271.

Torry, E. Fuller. 1988. *Nowhere to Go: The Tragic Odyssey of the Homeless Mentally Ill.* New York: Harper & Row.

Totterdell, Peter and David Holman. 2003. "Emotion Regulation in Customer Service Roles: Testing a Model of Emotional Labor." *Journal of Occupational Health Psychology* 8: 55–73.

Treweek, Geraldine L. 1996. "Emotion Work: Order, and Emotional Power in Care Assistant Work." Pp. 159–172 in *Health and the Sociology of Emotions*, edited by V. James and J. Gabe. Oxford, England: Blackwell Publishers.

Trice, Harrison M. 1993. *Occupational Subcultures in the Workplace*. Ithaca, NY: ILR Press.

————, and Janice M. Beyer. 1993. *The Cultures of Work Organizations*. Engelwood Cliffs, NJ: Prentice-Hall.

Tsui, Anne S. 1990. "A Multiple-Constituency Model of Effectiveness: An Empirical Examination at the Human Resource Subunit Level." *Administrative Science Quarterly* 35: 458–483.

Tucker, David J., Joel A. C. Baum, Jitendra V. Singh. 1992. "The Institutional Ecology of Human Service Organizations." Pp. 47–72 in *Human Services as Complex Organizations*, edited by Y. Hasenfeld. Newbury Park, CA: Sage.

Turner, Bryan. 1987. *Medical Power and Social Knowledge*. London: Sage.

Turney, Howard M., and Patricia Conway. 2000. "Managed Mental Health Care: Implications for Social Work Practice and Social Work Education." *Journal of Family Social Work* 5: 5–19.

Tuttle, Gayle McCraken and Dianne Rush Woods. 1997. *The Managed Care Answer Book For Mental Health Professionals*. Bristol, PA: Brunner/Mazel Publishers.

U.S. Department of Health and Human Services. 1999. Mental Health: A Report of the Surgeon General. Washington, DC: US Governmental Printing Office.

Van Maanen, John and Gideon Kunda. 1989. "'Real Feelings': Emotional Expression and Organizational Culture." Pp. 42–93 in *Research in Organizational Behavior*, edited by L. L. Cummings and B. M. Staw. Greenwich, CT: JAI Press.

Videka-Sherman, Lynn. 1988. "A Meta-analysis of Research on Social Work Practices in Mental Health." *Social Work* 33: 325–338.

Wagenfeld, M., and S. S. Robin. 1976. "Boundary Busting in the Community Mental Health Center." *Journal of Health and Social Behavior* 17: 112–122.

Wahl, Otto. 1995. *Media Madness*. New Brunswick, NJ: Rutgers University Press.

Wallace, J. E., and M. B. Brinkeroff. 1991. "The Measurement of Burnout Revisited." *Journal of Social Service Research* 14: 85–111.

Ware, Norma C., William S. Lachiocotte, Suzanne R. Kirschner, Dharma E. Cortes, and Byron J. Good. 2000. "Clinician Experiences of Managed Mental Health: A Rereading of the Threat." *Medical Anthropology Quarterly* 14: 3–27.

Warren, Mary Guptill, Rose Weitz, and Stephen Kulis. 1998. "Physician Satisfaction in a Changing Health Care Environment: The Impact of Challenges to Professional Autonomy, Authority, and Dominance." *Journal of Health and Social Behavior* 39: 356–367.

Waters, Malcolm. 1989. "Collegiality, Bureaucratization, and Professionalization: A Weberian Analysis." *American Journal of Sociology* 94: 945–972.

Weber, Max. 1946. *From Max Weber: Essays in Sociology*, edited and translated by H. H. Gerth and C. W. Mills. Oxford University Press.

Weick, Karl E. 1977. "Enactment Processes in Organizations." Pp. 267–300 in *New Directions in Organizational Behavior*, edited by B. M. Staw and G. Salancik. Chicago: St. Clair Press.

———. 1979. *The Social Psychology of Organizing*, 2nd ed. Reading, MA: Addison-Wesley.

——— and Richard L. Daft. 1983. "The Effectiveness of Interpretation Systems." Pp. 71–93 in *Organizational Effectiveness*, edited by K. S. Cameron and S. A. Whetton. New York: Academic Press.

Weiss, Marjorie and Ray Fitzpatrick. 1997. "Challenges to Medicine: The Case of Prescribing." *Sociology of Health and Illness*. 19: 297–327.

Weissman, E., K. Pettigre, S. Stosky and D. A. Regier. 2000. "The Cost of Access to Mental Health Services in Managed Care." *Psychiatric Services* 51: 664–66.

Wells, K. B., B. M. Astrachan, G. L. Tischer, and J. Unutzer. 1995. "Issues and Approaches in Evaluating Managed Mental Health Care." *The Milibank Quarterly* 73: 57–72.

Wharton, Amy S. 1993. "The Affective Consequences of Service Work: Managing Emotions on the Job." *Work and Occupations* 20: 205–232.

———, and Rebecca J. Erickson. 1995. "The Consequences of Caring: Exploring the Links Between Women's Job and Family Emotion Work." *The Sociological Quarterly* 36: 272–296.

Wiener, Carolyn L., and Jeanie Kayser-Jones. 1990. "The Uneasy Fate of Nursing Home Residents: An Organizational Interaction Perspective." *Sociology of Health and Illness* 12: 84–104.

Williams, Carol A. 1989. "Empathy and Burnout in Male and Female Helping Professions." *Research in Nursing and Health* 12: 169–178.

Williams, Simon. 1987. "Goffman, Interactionism, and the Management of Stigma in Everyday Life." Pp. 135–164 in *Sociological Theory and Medical Sociology*, edited by Graham Scambler. London: Tavistock Publications.

Wilson, Mitchell. 1993. "DSM-III and the Transformation of American Psychiatry." *American Journal of Psychiatry* 150: 399–410.

Wilson, Richard. 1992. *Compliance Ideologies: Rethinking Political Culture*. Cambridge, MA: Cambridge University Press.

Wolinksy, Frederic D. 1993. "The Professional Dominance, Deprofessionalization, Proletarianization, and Corporatization Perspectives: An Overview." Pp. 1–11 in *The Changing Medical Profession: An International Perspective*, edited by Frederic W. Hafferty and John B. McKinlay. New York: Oxford University Press.

Wolpin, Jacob, Ronald J. Burke, and Esther R. Greenglass. 1991. "Is Job Stress an Antecedent or Consequence of Psychological Burnout?" *Human Relations* 44: 193–209.

Wouters, Cas. 1989. "Commentary: The Sociology of Emotions and Flight Attendants: Hochschild's 'Managed Heart.'" *Theory, Culture and Society* 6: 95–123.

Wright, Peter, and Andrew Treacher. 1982. *The Problem of Medical Knowledge: Examining the Social Construction of Medicine*. Edinburgh, UK: Edinburgh University Press.

Yates, Brian T. 1996. *Analyzing Costs, Procedures, Processes and Outcomes in Human Services*. Newbury Park: Sage.

Zaph, Dieter, Claudia Seifert, Barbara Schmutte, Heidrun Mertini, and Melanie Holz. 2001. "Emotion Work and Job Stressors and Their Effect on Burnout." *Psychology and Health* 16: 527–545.

Zeitz, Gerald. 1983. "Structural and Individual Determinants of Organization Morale and Satisfaction." *Social Forces* 61: 1088–1108.

Ziengenfuss, James T. 1983. *Patients Rights and Organizational Models: Sociotechnical Systems Reseasrch on Mental Health Programs*. Washington, DC: University Press.

Zucker, Lynne G. 1987. "Institutional Theories of Organization." *Annual Review of Sociology* 13: 443–464.

Index

Abbott, Andrew, 3–5, 42
Accountability and managed care, 162, 166
Adjustment as goal of treatment, 47–48, 50, 52
Advocacy efforts of mental health care providers, 4, 151–153
Agency for Healthcare Research and Quality, 145
Aiken, Linda H., 79, 108
American Psychological Association, 25
"Analytical examination of medical work," 2
Any-willing provider (AWP), 153
Ashforth, Blake E., 110–111
Assertive Community Treatment (ACT), 33, 43
Assertive Treatment Technical Assistance Center, 151
Asylums (Goffman), 44
Autonomy
  for client, 50
  as goal of treatment, 47–49
  labor management and, 134
  mental health care providers and, 86, 95, 158

Bazelton Center for Mental Health Law, 141–142, 147–148, 152–153
"Behavioral health care" organizations, 67
Beigel, Allan, 63, 139
Ben-Dror, Raphael, 84
Benner, Patricia, 15, 45
Biomedical perspective of treatment, 3, 8, 24–28, 33
Biopsychosocial perspective of treatment, 34–37, 157
Birne-Stone, Susan, 78

Black, Bruce L., 36
Boys in White (study), 2
British National Health Service, 125
Buck, Jeffrey A., 67
Bureaucratic model of organizations, 63
Bureaucratization
  incompatibility of, with mental health care, 164–165
  managed care and, 79, 86–89, 159, 162
  of mental health care provider, 86–89, 158
  of nursing home care, 4
Burfoot, Jean, 108, 121
Burke, A. C., 46
Burke, Ronald, 105
Burnout in mental health care (*see also* Emotional labor)
  CARE and, 105, 112–118, 130–132, 138, 160–161
  causal analysis of, 136
  client demands and, 108, 155
  context of, 13
  defining, 11–12
  emotional demands and, 110
  emotional labor and, 12–13, 105–106, 122
  empathy and, 107–108
  etiology of, 108, 122
  implications for, 137–138
  literature on, 2
  managed care and, 130, 159–160
  Maslach Burnout Inventory and, 107
  mental health care work and, 12
  Ordinary Least Squares regression analysis of, 135–136
  organizational conditions and, 13, 108, 136, 155, 159
  overburdened providers and, 137–138
  overview, 108–109

For Product Safety Concerns and Information please contact our EU
representative GPSR@taylorandfrancis.com Taylor & Francis Verlag GmbH,
Kaufingerstraße 24, 80331 München, Germany

Printed and bound by CPI Group (UK) Ltd, Croydon, CR0 4YY
08/06/2025
01897011-0006